My Doctor Never Told Me That!

My Doctor Never Told Me That!

Things you always wanted to know about your health...
without all the technical MUMBO JUMBO

CHRISTINE SPURLOCK, D.C.
MADISON SPURLOCK, D.C.

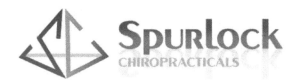

www.spurlockchiropractic.com

New York

My Doctor Never Told me That!

Things you always wanted to know about your health…
without all the technical MUMBO JUMBO

ISBN 978-1-60037-689-4

Library of Congress Control Number: 2009933975

MORGAN · JAMES
THE ENTREPRENEURIAL PUBLISHER

Morgan James Publishing, LLC
1225 Franklin Ave., STE 325
Garden City, NY 11530-1693
Toll Free 800-485-4943
www.MorganJamesPublishing.com

Note to reader: This book is intended as an informational guide. The remedies, approaches, and techniques described herein are meant to supplement, and not to be a substitute for, professional medical care or treatments. They should not be used to treat a serious ailment without prior consultation with a qualified health-care professional.

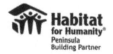

In an effort to support local communities, raise awareness and funds, Morgan James Publishing donates one percent of all book sales for the life of each book to Habitat for Humanity. Get involved today, visit **www.HelpHabitatForHumanity.org.**

This book is dedicated to Pooh and Fee,
the twinkle in our eyes and reason to rise.
~P. & C.

Smart People Make Smart Patients

Give a man a fish and feed him for a day; teach a man to fish and feed him for a lifetime.

Chiropractors play a vital role in the communities they serve, providing relief through simple, effective adjustments that take away pain and restore peace of mind. But the work doesn't stop there. Because life in a community is a give-and-take experience, those with knowledge to share have a responsibility to spread the word to enhance the quality of life for everyone.

We take great pride in the role we perform as small-town chiropractors. We recognize the unique opportunity we have to enrich the lives in our community—by our actions *and* our words. Our training has made us aware of the remarkable connections that allow our bodies to function as they do. It has also made us understand how dysfunctions can occur. This knowledge is enabling us to treat the people who come to us for help.

But our knowledge can be used in other ways, too. By stepping outside the confines of the clinic and sharing the underlying "why" that lies beneath the pain, we have the ability to educate our existing patients and our patients yet to come … giving them a better understanding of the influences that shape their world, their relationships, and their mental, physical, and emotional health. We have the ability to enable them to make smart choices now and in the future.

- Awareness is step one in the process of change.
- Belief is step two.
- Commitment is step three.

Our purpose in creating this educational opportunity and sharing it with you is to provide you with the tools to make the smart, informed choices that will enrich your lives.

The 120 articles that follow are grouped into three sections and multiple categories. Each article provides a nugget of information that allows you to make simple adjustments in your daily lives. These adjustments are part of a program of awareness treatments designed to begin the healing process of change and give you a quality of life you deserve.

We are dedicated to long-term health and wellness. As we share our knowledge with you and you pass on the benefits to the people you love, our industry takes a valued step forward.

Thank you for joining our chiropractic family.

Christine and Madison Spurlock

Table of Contents

SECTION ONE: THE BIG, WIDE WORLD 1

Chapter One: Science 3
Chapter Two: Tools & Technology 13
Chapter Three: We're not Alone! 25
Chapter Four: Food, Glorious Food 39

SECTION TWO: HOW WE COPE ... AND DON'T! 59

Chapter One: Reactions 61
Chapter Two: Conditions & Syndromes. 86
Chapter Three: Behaviors 109
Chapter Four: Diseases. 138
Chapter Five: Viruses & Allergies. 148
Chapter Six: Pregnancy 160
Chapter Seven: Hormones 168
Chapter Eight: Energy Imbalances 176

SECTION THREE: THE MAGNIFICENT MIRACLE 185

Chapter One: Systems 187
Chapter Two: Organs. 211
Chapter Three: Skin. 219
Chapter Four: Muscles 232
Chapter Five: Nerves 238
Chapter Six: Joints 247
Chapter Seven: Bones. 265

About the Authors. 273

SECTION ONE:
THE BIG, WIDE WORLD

A physician is obligated to consider more than a diseased organ, more even than the whole man— he must view the man in his world.

~Harvey Cushing

We never step in the same river twice ... because the river is always moving and we are always changing. As we change and grow, the world changes, too, and these changes bring with them exciting new advances and opportunities.

We ready ourselves to adjust to these changes on many levels ... preparing our minds and our bodies to adopt new practices and adapt to new influences that we have never known before.

To make the most of these opportunities, we need to know the risks and understand our responsibilities in order to enjoy the rewards.

The articles in this section are intended to provide a guide as you follow this path and experience the world around you.

- Chapter 1 talks about scientific discoveries;
- Chapter 2 introduces tools and technology;
- Chapter 3 reminds us that we're not alone;
- Chapter 4 is all about food, glorious food!

Chapter One:
Science

The deviation of man from the state in which he was originally placed by nature seems to have proved to him a prolific source of disease.

– Edward Jenner

Cryonics: The Art of People Popsicles

Ever hear about someone falling into an icy lake and living through it? Sometimes they make it even after an hour or two without oxygen. This miracle seems to defy everything we've learned about our need for warmth and air.

What happens is that when the body gets put on ice it goes into "suspended animation" mode. This slows everything to a pace at which the brain needs almost no oxygen. With cryonics, someone who is legally dead is placed into liquid nitrogen and kept frozen for years. This is a little on the creepy side for a lot of people, and no, I have no plans to become a human Popsicle. But creepy can be interesting, so let's take a look at the nuts and bolts of the cryonics process.

So how does it work? Are they just placed into freezers? Not so simple. First you have to be a member of a cryonic facility. (Dues are around $400 a year.) After you are declared legally dead, the response team springs into action. While being transported to the facility, they supply your brain with oxygen and blood. Your blood is also given an anticoagulant to keep it from clotting. At the facility, more tinkering has to be done because we are largely comprised of water. The problem is that when water freezes, it expands. (That's why you never leave a can of anything in the freezer.) This expansion would ultimately cause all your cells to shatter, so they take all the water out of your cells and put *cryoprotectant* in its place. This acts like human anti-freeze, keeping ice crystals from forming. Finally, the body is immersed head down (to save the brain in case it springs a leak) in a vat of liquid nitrogen. Just to add to the creepiness factor, each storage tank holds four full bodies. At least you're not alone, right?

The theory behind cryonics is that the freezing process will be reversed, and you'll be toasted up sometime after the disease you've lived with is cured. I know what you're thinking: "What about that other problem, being dead and all?" You're right; that's a toughie. According to loyal cryonics followers, there are hairs to split here. They do their work when a patient is *legally* dead, meaning no heartbeat. It's not the same as *totally* dead, which is when there is no brain activity.

How much green would this run you? It's about $150,000 for a whole body. Looking for a discount? A neurosuspension (just your brain) is $50K. The projected timetable most cryonics labs have is the year 2040 for the first defrosting. This is their best guess as to the time when medical breakthroughs will have found cures and our technologies will achieve success. The frozen crowd has at least one celebrity among its ranks: baseball legend Ted Williams has been on ice since his death in 2002. His body is in Arizona in a luxury singleton tank.

Maybe it's just me, but to wake in another world without the ones you love might feel more like a nightmare. I say spend your time appreciating today and let your children have tomorrow.

Just What the Doctor Ordered?

Medical errors kill more Americans than car accidents, breast cancer, and AIDS combined, yet there are no marches, bracelets, or ribbons worn proudly on protesters' chests. Outside medical circles, it's not a topic that's brought up very much. This is a shame, because the best way to prevent a medical error is to be proactive in your care and make yourself aware of the possible pitfalls. Medical professionals are doing what they can, but you have to do your part, too.

Let's take a look inside the doctor's office and get up close and personal with the medicines she prescribes. Is it just what the doctor ordered? With prescriptions, sometimes the answer is yes and sometimes it's no. If you can't make heads or tails of your prescription, who says that your pharmacist can? Pharmacists have no secret radar vision that lets them know what your doctor really meant to prescribe. So take action and ask your doctor to clearly print the name of the drug if you can't read it.

Knowing when to take the medication and how much is not enough. You should also ask for an explanation of possible side effects. This will help you know what to look out for and what risks you might face.

It's also smart to "brown bag" it when you go for your checkup. Don't just tell your physician what meds you are on; show him or her what you've got. Take all your meds, supplements, and vitamins with you. Drug names have crazy spellings, and they also have pertinent information, like dosages and compatibilities, right on the bottle.

Another good practice is to remind your physician if you are pregnant, breastfeeding, or have a preexisting condition, such as diabetes, before your prescription is written. These conditions can make a difference, and the doctor will thank you for saving valuable time. It also pays to bring someone with you to your appointment—someone you don't mind sharing your personal medical information with. An extra set of ears can help you remember all the instructions. Your friend or family member can also help you remember your own health history.

Write down all of your symptoms and questions before your appointment. You may think you won't forget, but you may only have a few minutes together. When you're dealing with all the questions your doctor may have, plus the tests and measurements taken, it's easy to get sidetracked, and important items can get forgotten.

No news is not always good news. If you had a test taken, find out the results. Don't just assume that you will get a call. Even the best professionals can get overloaded and forget to pick up the phone. Always know that "more" is not always better. Ask if a test or treatment is really needed and how it would help you. You might be better off without it or have other options available.

Listen to your inner voice. Pay attention to your body and the things it is telling you. If you listen to the whispers, the body may not have to yell. Make yourself a priority and invite others to treat you as one.

Stem Cells: A Fresh Start?

Stem-cell research, all of us have heard of it. Most of us know it's controversial, and a number have our minds made up about it. But, beyond the hype and headlines, very few of us know what it actually is. So before we state that we're for or against this cause, let's try to decipher the code.

We have 220 different varieties of cells in our bodies. Some come together to make up our organs, while others are busy forming our bones, skin, and everything else in between. What they all have in common is that, once upon a time, they were all stem cells.

Three to five days after conception, all that we will become is contained with some 100 cells that together are no bigger than the period at the end of this sentence. These are the embryonic stem cells. They are unique, because they can become any type of cell. Science calls these cells *de*differentiated. This unique ability to grow into any other type of cell is what makes them so important and why scientists are making such a fuss. But this versatility is a one-time thing. Once they have taken the path of becoming a specific cell, they can't change again and be anything different.

Adult stem cells have not been as popular because, until recently, it was believed that these cells were set in their ways; that an adult stem cell from bone marrow could only make more marrow; that adult stem cells in our lungs and other organs could only produce more of the same organ- specific cells. The good news is that research now suggests that they may have more flexibility.

Whether it is adult or embryonic, what is all the fuss about? The thinking is that scientists may be able to grow a specific type of stem cell and then inject it into a specific tissue. By placing new cardiac tissue in someone who had a heart attack—or introducing nerve tissue in someone whose spine has been severed—it is hoped that healthy new tissue would eventually take over and replace the damaged tissue.

It sounds pretty far-fetched, but it's not such a distant leap of faith. These experiments have already been done successfully on rats. In a Mayo study, rats that suffered heart attacks had rodent stem cells injected into their hearts. Eventually, the stem cells took over and replaced the scarred cardiac muscle tissue.

Since the 1960s, stem-cell transplants—more commonly known as bone-marrow transplants—have successfully been treating human patients with leukemia.

This journey is not without difficult choices and technical challenges. Before they can safely and ethically recommend their use, scientists need to be sure that the stem cells injected into a liver will become liver cells and not make a wrong turn and grow into bone cells, for example, or something else. Scientists also need to know that they will stop growing at the right time and not become a tumor or migrate to another part of the body and do something unwelcome there.

With stem-cell research, the stakes are high. The ethical debate is a heated one. It is hopeful that adult stem cells may be more of a viable resource than once believed. This could help us all find more common ground whose benefits could be life saving.

Who Is the WHO?

Ever hear of the WHO? I'm not talking about the band, though they'd be an interesting topic some other time. No, the WHO I'm referring to is the World Health Organization. We've all heard some tidbit that started out as, "According to the World Health Organization ...." But what exactly is it that makes the WHO such a big deal? We're citizens of the world, so we should know what they are doing on our behalf, right? Right!

The World Health Organization was born on April 7, 1948, which we now celebrate every year as World Health Day. You probably don't get this day off work yet, which is why it may have gone unnoticed until now. The WHO was the brainchild of the League of Nations and was later adopted by the United Nations. The main hub is in Switzerland and has representatives from governments from around the globe. Most of the big decisions happen during their main meeting at the beginning of each year.

With many lofty goals, the WHO has its work cut out for it. Its stated reason for being is, "to aid in the attainment of the highest possible level of health by all people." Not too shabby. By health, they mean, "a state of complete physical, mental, and social well-being and not merely the absence of disease or infirmity." Needless to say, they have a long way to go.

How does the WHO go about getting all this done? They're involved in everything from health education to sanitation to the prevention and control of diseases. They're behind the drive to coordinate a global strategy to control the spread of AIDS. The WHO promotes the sharing of information as well. In a world where a bug can hitch a ride and go globetrotting in a matter of days, this spirit of shared communication is essential.

In its sixty-year history, the WHO has done a lot of good. A huge success story for the organization is the eradication of smallpox, which was as big a threat in its time as AIDS is today. No one can deny the relevance of that accomplishment: smallpox is the only human infectious disease to have been completely eradicated. In spite of its achievements, the WHO has its share of critics. Just like any giant organization, the WHO is often overwhelmed by its red tape. Harsh criticisms have sprung up against its tobacco control measures and compulsory vaccinations, for example.

The issue the objections circle around is freedom of choice. There will always be people who resist change, despite tangible proof that change is an essential component for species survival and growth. The WHO's aim is for us to reach our highest level of health. Hopefully that's a personal goal for all of us, too.

Electromagnetic Waves: The New Air Pollution

Research shows that electrical pollution is killing us. Researchers fear overhead power lines, airwave communication, florescent lights, computers, and even hair dryers and other electrical appliances are affecting our health. The problem lies in the fact that potentially harmful electromagnetic fields run on alternating current, while our own energy fields and nervous systems run on direct current. Whether you call it chi, aura, or life force, our electromagnetic energy is the essential to life itself.

In a sense, our energy field acts as a front line of defense, repelling harmful things in our environment. You know how it feels when you try to push the same pole sides of two magnets together. You can't see the force at work resisting your efforts, but you sure can feel the energy that continues to keep those poles apart. This energy force is how we repel negative energies that try to attack us. The problem occurs when there is a breakdown or weakness in our magnetic field and we lose that defensive ability. Our energy field ends up looking like Swiss cheese, allowing things to pass through.

Dr. William Philpott (*New Hope for Physical and Emotional Illness*) states his opinion that many human diseases and discomforts are caused by an imbalance of North Pole and South Pole energies in each cell. When the North Pole energy is weakened, arterial blood becomes more acidic. Viruses, parasites, and other pathogenic organisms grow in an acidic environment. North Pole magnetic energy raises the pH of the blood, making it more alkaline, thus reducing the overgrowth of disease-causing organisms.

Many people feel weak, have headaches, or feel unwell when they work in front of computers or under florescent lights. Carpal tunnel was quite rare when old manual typewriters were used, yet it has become increasingly common in people using new, easy to push, computer keyboards.

Try this test. Stand and put your arm straight out in front of you. Have someone push down on your arm and see how strong it is. Then do the same exercise again while standing close to a computer or TV set that is turned on. You'll probably find that your arm becomes quite weak. The only variable that has changed is your proximity to electric alternating currents.

Even though we can't do away with these electrical bombardments, we can protect ourselves. Therapeutic multipolar magnets no bigger than a credit card have been found to be very effective in many types of conditions, including chronic pain, headaches, carpal tunnel, tennis elbow, strained muscles, bruises, arthritis, back pain, and spinal problems. At our office, we use the test mentioned above and retest with the patient holding the magnet. In most cases, the patient will be noticeably stronger right away.

Regular magnets won't work, so don't bother with the one stuck to your refrigerator. It must be a multipolar magnet, which means that the North-South poles alternate in strips. It must be rated at a *gauss* (the measurement for electromagnetic fields) that is in the low organic range of 1–4s. More is not better, and having a magnet too strong will have adverse effects. There are many types of multipolar magnets on the market that are suitable, and the prices vary.

Chapter Two:
Tools & Technology

We are living in a world today where lemonade is made from artificial flavors and furniture polish is made from real lemons.

~Alfred E. Newman

Air Fresheners: Pollution You Can Plug In

Who doesn't want their home to smell like pumpkin spice or freshly baked apple pie? The very thought makes the mouth water, doesn't it? The problem is we'd have to be baking these goodies all the time to keep that beautiful aroma blowing around the home.

Thanks to the good folks at companies that make air fresheners, we don't have to spend our days in the kitchen to create those tantalizing fragrances any more. All we have to do is "plug it in," and our homes are homey without all the work.

Unfortunately, this deal is less than sweet. These gadgets are dispensing a lot more than you think. Along with familiar aromas, they're spewing out pollution and putting our lives at risk.

To be technically correct, air fresheners should be called "air covers." They don't actually suck up the smell wafting over the trash or Fido's bad breath. They just cover it with a "better" smell. The problem is that these covers are chemically engineered and come in the form of volatile chemicals called *pinene* and *limonene*. How volatile, you ask? At high levels, they have been shown to promote cancer.

Of course, air fresheners only release tiny amounts of these chemicals, so you could say that they pose just a tiny risk of causing cancer. Yikes. If that weren't reason enough to unplug, when the emissions from air fresheners are combined with ozone, the result is formaldehyde: a chemical that can trigger asthma and other nasty respiratory problems. Ozone can come from outdoor pollution, but it is also found in bleach and in sterilization agents for air and drinking water. At low concentrations, it is toxic. Even in rural areas, prevailing winds can blow pollutants our way, making it a health hazard as serious for us as it is for Mother Earth.

And one more cautionary note: plug-in air fresheners have been cited as the cause of enough house fires to prompt the voluntary recall of the extra outlet variety due to this risk. So let's clear the air once and for all. Air fresheners emit chemicals that have been proven, at higher rates, to cause cancer. Check. They can trigger asthma. Check. They can burn down your house. Check. Do they actually clear the air and remove stinky stuff? Nope. When you add up the results, Fido's breath doesn't seem so bad after all.

Sometimes there is truly nothing like the real thing. A floral fragrance is much sweeter coming from a bouquet of flowers, and when you walk into a home filled with the smell of freshly baked apple pie, it's much nicer to know that America's favorite homemade dessert is on its way.

Can the Boob Tube Cause Autism?

Ahhh, the TV: the greatest unpaid babysitter there is. That box in the corner that our lives are centered around. All our furniture stands grouped around it. Mealtimes are scheduled to coincide with favorite shows. TV specials are occasions to invite friends over to celebrate. On ordinary nights, we spend hours flipping channels with that handy device we call the remote.

We could criticize television for its endless commercials. We could also talk about the link to obesity, but more important to talk about right now are the findings from a recent study linking the boob tube to an increase in autism in our children. Autism rates have been on the rise, along with the number of parents searching for answers.

What is autism? For those who saw the Tom Cruise/Dustin Hoffman film, *Rain Man*, the image of a disconnected, dysfunctional individual is very clear. But the condition has many faces. Two children with autism can be totally different in the severity and challenges placed before them.

In most cases, there is a difficulty in connecting with others. This can be the child who does not look you in the eye or, when shown a picture of a baby in a toy car, is much more interested in the car. Children with autism will often feel safe in their rituals. They will not want you to wrap your arms around them. It can take some guesswork, but with care, autism can even be diagnosed as early as toddlerhood.

What causes autism? One theory is that the mercury from vaccinations could be the culprit. Vaccine companies have denied this, meanwhile removing the mercury from most of their products. Television is also falling under scrutiny, thanks to researchers from Cornell and Purdue, who have found that autism levels rose in direct proportion to the prevalence of cable TV in our homes. They also noted that autism rates were higher in rainier parts of the country.

What does this all mean and why is rain a factor? The cable TV theory suggests that for children who watch excessive amounts of TV before the age of three, it can "trigger" autism, meaning that for toddlers who are straddling the fence on autism, TV can become the straw that breaks this camel's back. As for the rain factor, children tend to spend more time inside with the electronic babysitter when it rains.

This study does not deliver a definitive cause/effect indicator. What it does best is open up the dialogue to other possibilities. It also reminds us of something we already know: that it's good to play and give the TV a rest when you can.

You might consider angling your furniture to create conversational groupings that include the TV without giving it a place of honor. You never know: you might meet someone interesting and learn something really new.

The Cell Phone and Your Brain

Have you tried telling your grandchildren you remember a time before the cell phone, before the days of rollover minutes, ring tones, and all the cute little accessories? If you have, I'm sure they looked at you in the same way you looked at your grandparents when they talked about life before electricity, indoor plumbing, and the automobile. Like, how primitive!

Cell phones are such a bread-and-butter part of our lives now that it's hard to remember how we managed without them. It won't be long before the antiquated pay phone and traditional car phone will be headed for the scrap yard. The question is, do our cell phones love us back? Are they expanding our circle or quietly shutting down our brains? Let's look at the controversy and try to answer the questions about the cell phone's impact on our health.

Let's start with a lesson—we'll call it Radiation 101. "Electromagnetic radiation" is the term that describes waves of electric and magnetic energy traveling at the speed of light. The waves we get from our cell phones are in the same neighborhood as the radiation from a microwave.

This type of *nonionizing radiation* is classified as *relatively* safe. But unlike our exposure in front of the microwave when we nuke a snack or heat up accompaniments for a meal, we are holding these radiating gadgets up to our precious noggins for hours a day. And just like a microwave heats food, this radiation heats up our brain. A rate of 1.6 watts per kilogram (of human tissue) is the acceptable limit, according to experts. How do we know how many watts we're getting? And how do we know how accurate these "experts" are?

"If cell phone were at all dangerous, they'd be illegal, right?" Everyone assumes that someone is looking out for our best interests. But it wasn't that long ago that cigarettes weren't considered harmful beyond the occasional throat irritation from excessive smoke. It took years of research and mountains of money to discover the truth. On the upside, the FCC requires every cell phone model to be tested for "overall heating effect of radio-frequency energy." The downside is that they let the manufacturers conduct the tests themselves.

So the questions are beginning to form. Do we have a conflict of interest issue here? Will the effects from long-term cell phone use be revealed anytime soon? Where will they find the guinea pigs to use for their study groups?

Since we are the first generation to use the cell phone like an extension of our selves, we are the study group. And it will be at least another ten years until the dust finally settles and we know the results. Until then, we're not advocating a ban on cell phones altogether, and fortunately this is not an all-or-nothing issue. We have a number of alternatives available to us. We can follow our European counterparts. In the UK, the Ministry of Health advised all children and pregnant women not to use cell phones. In more and more states, a hands-free device is mandatory when driving, and these units establish a healthy distance between the radiation and your brain. In many cities, cell phone use is prohibited in public places.

We also advise that you limit your time talking in enclosed spaces. Weather permitting, take a step outside for a breath of fresh air before you reach out and touch someone. Remember that, as with most things, cell phones are not created equally. Check the FCC Web page list for radiation outputs for different models.

And remember that it's okay to enjoy being in the moment. Sometimes a walk or a drive is a great time to enjoy the silence and celebrate your own quiet thoughts.

Hearing Loss: Music to Your Ears?

Have you noticed that the comfort volume on your TV is creeping up? Is it getting harder to hear your partner nowadays?

Hearing loss can happen so gradually that it's easy to blame it on hushed voices. It can come from many sources, but one of the most common is loud noises. New gadgets come with new concerns, so we'll give some special attention to MP3 players, including iPods, as we look at ways we can protect our hearing.

These personal players have improved on the old Walkman in so many ways: they're smaller, they hold and play a bazillion songs, and the music is much crisper. That's all to the good, right? Maybe not. The hidden safety feature of the Walkman was its limited range of volume. If you tried to turn it up too high, all you got was static. People ended up negotiating a volume level that was loud enough to hear and still understand the words that were sung. Now that this barrier has been overcome, we are left to set our own limits. In addition, with so many songs on our playlists, we're listening much longer. Time will only tell how much damage we are doing. So until then, try to be gentle to your ears.

"Wait," you're saying. "How does hearing loss happen, anyway?" It's pretty simple, really. You have tiny little hairs in your inner ear that sprout from the cells in your cochlea. Their job is to act like tiny antennae and capture the sounds all around them. What causes damage is when the sound waves are so powerful that these little hairs are knocked over. After a rock concert, you might say that these little guys have a bad hair day, which translates into temporary damage. Until they recover—it usually takes a couple of days—familiar sounds often seem muffled, or you might hear a buzzing sound in place of the silence you usually enjoy.

Permanent hearing loss can come from one really loud noise, such as a gunshot, that flattens the hairs so completely that they never recover. It can also come from consistent exposure to moderately loud noises over time. This is where MP3 and iPod use come in, and where car stereos cranked to the max do the harm.

What is considered a dangerous level of sound? Let's talk decibels. Any noise over ninety decibels can eventually cause hearing loss. When cranked all the way up, most MP3 players and iPods can reach 120 decibels. That's as loud as an ambulance siren, by the way, or the sound of a jet aircraft taking off. Ouch! Just as every car needs seatbelts and every computer has some type of spam/antivirus program, we need to take precautions with our toys. Protect your ears and turn it down. You want to be able to enjoy the silence when it comes.

Nasal Sprays: Some People Just Can't Get Enough

Are you addicted to your nasal spray? Can you get addicted to it? Sitting in its cute little bottle with no prescription needed, it can't really become a crutch, can it? With runny nose season becoming a year-round event, we need to get to the bottom of this misty wonder. Let's figure out what decongestant nasal spray actually is and find out when it's better to just sweat it out.

Nasal sprays don't make you do harmful or crazy things, and they don't stimulate the pleasure center in the brain, which means that it's not likely that anyone is going to steal from Grandma's sock drawer to score some nasal spray. However, the fact that they are not addictive by scientific or medical standards doesn't mean we can let these sprays off the hook just yet.

What nasal sprays are guilty of promoting is something called "rebound congestion," which is a way of saying that they can eventually cause more problems than they cure. But before we get into how they don't work, let's go over what they're supposed to do.

Decongestant nasal sprays work by constricting the blood vessels in your nose. No matter if your sniffles come from a cold, the flu, or a reaction to Fido's fur, the blood vessels in your nose will become swollen or dilated. This triggers your nasal membranes to work overtime and make a surplus crop of gooey mucus. People find this mess inconvenient and reach for a nasal spray because, with a simple magic squirt or two, the leaky faucet is shut off.

Now this is where these sprays can overstay their welcome. After a few days, the body gets wise and launches a counterattack. Your nose seriously dilates your blood vessels, canceling out the effect the spray once had. To get the same relief, you're stuck spraying more and more.

Your nose and the spray are stuck in a dysfunctional relationship, each one upping the ante until your fingers get sore and rebound congestion is born. Is an amicable split possible here? Not without a little heartbreak, which comes in the form of going "cold turkey" and putting up with congestion for periods of a month and more until your body gets back to normal.

The thing to remember before you start is that nasal sprays are not meant for long-term use. When your nose runs, think twice before you run out to the drugstore and consider some of the natural choices out there ... like taking vitamins to boost your immune system, breathing in the warm vapors of hot apple cider vinegar, keeping the house free of dust and other pollutants, and getting enough rest. If none of that works for you, there's always the old-fashioned way of letting your body do the job it was meant to do while you grab a hanky and collect sympathy points.

Heavy Metal: Is It in You?

Many of us remember experiments from high school chemistry class ... those beakers, some unlucky frog, and a thermometer filled with mercury. If some klutz broke the thermometer, it was cleaned up carefully so no one touched the toxic substance or breathed in its fumes.

We take those precautions with all heavy metals, right? Wrong. The fact is, many of us ingest them, breathe them in, and even roll them on our underarms without a second thought. So let's talk about the heavy metals that find their way into our systems and learn how to run them off.

Our industrialized nation has put metals in our medicine cabinets and refrigerators. Most vaccinations still contain mercury. Those shiny fillings in our mouths are made of some sort of metallic mixture. But this is just the tip of the iceberg. We've taken the lead out of paint, but it's still in makeup and some hair coloring. Nickel is found in hydrogenated oils, chocolate, and in some drinking water. Aluminum is used in baking powder, processed cheese, and antiperspirants.

People often wonder why aluminum is used in antiperspirants. Aluminum is a charged ion. When you roll or spray on antiperspirant, the metal gets sucked up into the cells in your armpit. Water, which is already in your system, soon follows the aluminum, causing the cells to swell up. In no time, the cells are so swollen no water can get in or out. When the body disperses the intruder, another application is needed.

So what's the big deal? What's the problem with having a little extra chrome in our ride? Some studies point to a link to autism and Alzheimer's. Mercury can cause headaches, skin rashes, and poor mental concentration. Nickel can cause allergies. Symptoms of metal in your system can be anything from muscle weakness to constant wheezing.

No amount of toxic heavy metals is good for you, yet it's one of the last things we'd point a finger at.

You're never going to avoid all toxic metals, but making some conscious choices to avoid adding new metal to our bodies is a start. Read food labels. Reduce the quantity of processed foods in your diet. You don't need to stop using antiperspirants and go "all natural"; just buy deodorant without the sweat stopper.

The other part is getting those meddling metals that you do have, out. There are some good oral chelation supplements at most health food stores. You could also try a good ion footbath detoxification. It is important to work with your chiropractor or other experienced health-care providers when detoxing metals, because steps need to be taken not to go too fast. Also, taking the right supplements is important to get the metal out, not just stirred up in your system.

Sometimes the quest to good health may seem like a complicated journey—one in which outside guidance is needed. Applying a toxic metal to your bare skin every day probably doesn't sit well with your gut instincts. Trust that, and let it be your guide.

Chapter Three:
We're not Alone!

Life preys upon life. This is biology's most fundamental fact.

~Martin H. Fischer

"Friendly" Bacteria

"Don't touch that! It might have bacteria on it."
In a world that promotes antibacterial everything, it might seem that bacteria have become public enemy #1. Corporate America pushes soaps and sprays to keep those nasty little critters away. Antibiotics are given to our livestock to fight infection, and they're given to us directly from the prescription pad.

But did you know that not all bacteria are alike? Some bacteria—like the one that causes meningitis—can kill you, while others actually have an important job to do in the body. Without these friendly bacteria, we'd have a hard time digesting food. Let's shine a light on these bacteria, get to know who they are and what they do, and make it a dirty word no more.

For things to flow smoothly, we need billions of friendly bacteria floating around in our digestive systems. Are you having trouble imagining what billions of bacteria might look like? Think of four pounds spread out everywhere along the many miles of highways and byways inside you.

All in all, there are seven different types of healthy bacteria; each group is hard at work tackling particular tasks. You may not notice them when they are here, but when they're gone, your body certainly misses them. What exactly do these guys do? One kind keeps the level of yeast in your body in check. Another keeps you from getting gassy. Another is in cahoots with your immune system, keeping you healthy.

With all the antibacterial action we have going on outside, you're probably wondering how these friendly critters get past the guards and get inside. If you eat a well-balanced diet, they take up residence in our intestines.

What drives them away? Antibiotics do not discriminate. When you take them to kill off bad bacteria, they kill the good types, too. If you eat meat that's not organic, your healthy bacteria count may dwindle. Eating refined carbohydrates can send these good tenants packing, too.

If your population of good bacteria is not what it should be, what would that look like? For some it might be gas, indigestion, and bloating. For others, it could be yeast overgrowth. It can throw some peoples' hormones off balance or just make you feel generally unwell.

So if bacteria can be something your body wants because it can be helpful and not icky at all, how do we get it inside us … lick the bottom of a dirty shoe? I should hope not! To get good bacteria in your system, you can take *probiotics*. This word comes from the Greek, and it means "for life." Most natural health-care providers and stores carry them, and many commercially made brands of yogurt now promote them. Always take them on an empty stomach, as the acidity of the stomach during meals can damage some of these bacteria. A great way to start your day right is to take probiotics first thing. You can also get friendly bacteria from the foods you eat. Natural yogurt is a great source.

Finding balance for your body sometimes takes work, but it's much easier than living poorly.

Don't Let the Bed Bugs Bite

Remember your mom telling you there were no monsters hiding in the closet? She'd also look under the bed, making sure the coast was clear. Your eyes would close, and you'd drift away and dream. Good thing there's no such thing as big bad monsters, right?

Well, sometimes monsters come in pint-size packages, and if you've ever wakened with bed-bug bites, you know they can pack a powerful punch. These reddish brown creatures have six legs; the largest are smaller than a ladybug, and they work the night shift so you don't see them by day. The crime scene isn't particularly gory. A careful examination will turn up little more than tiny bloodstains on the sheets and mattress.

Where the real damage is done is on you. After you've been bitten, you have a large, itchy wheal on your skin. Sometimes you end up with groups of small, pus-filled sacs and rashes on your skin. To the creepiness factor, the room will have a sickly sweet smell from the bugs' oily secretions.

Chances are you didn't feel a thing as they clamped down. This is because they release an anesthetic to numb the site first. They also inject an anticoagulant, so your blood flows freely for them. Even worse, these critters are making a big comeback. What was once little more than a campfire story has become a world traveler, thanks to so many of us getting itchy feet and seeing the world. They're also growing in number because the chemical DDT is being used less often to kill bugs, ever since it was discovered that the chemical was harmful to humans, too.

So how do you win the battle against these midnight marauders? Your washing machine is your first line of defense, and things need to get hot in here. Bedding should be washed at 115 degrees to smoke them out. You should also inspect any secondhand furniture before you cart it home. When you go on vacation and check into your room, make sure you're bunking alone. Pull back the blankets and check out the sheet. If sanitary conditions are not up to snuff, don't be too shy to ask for another room.

The good news about bed-bug bites (if there could be) is that the bites usually heal on their own within a couple of weeks. While they're really itchy and not a subject you want to share with your hairdresser, they spread no diseases and have no lasting physical effects. I wish I could say the memory of these home wreakers could fade just as quickly.

Sleep tight and don't let the bed bugs bite.

Bird Flu: Why This Isn't Just for the Birds

We've heard about bird flu. We've seen pictures from somewhere in Asia or Eastern Europe of people in masks burning stockpiles of birds. If it's getting so much coverage, we imagine that it must be a big deal ... at least to the people who have to burn up their livelihoods. But we're safely tucked away in a country where healthy chickens abound. And even if this flu thing becomes a problem, our government will issue the vaccines to keep us safe and warm, right?

Not so fast. Today's mobile society is constantly on the move. With modern transportation systems making world travel affordable, we're visiting far-flung places all over the globe in record time. We're sharing our lives and lifestyles with others more than ever before.

So far, tens of millions of birds and dozens of people have died from the bird flu. In most cases, people have caught the virus directly from a sick bird. The story, which gets repeated, is that a bird with bird flu gives the disease to a human. This person is probably poor and sleeping under the same roof as the livestock. Officials isolate the person in a hospital and kill all local birds. In many cases, the person also dies. Tourism drops in that country, and many countries ban some imports from there. As sad as that is, that's not what keeps some people at the Centers for Disease Control and Prevention up at night. What worries them is the possibility of the bird flu spreading from person to person. If this happens, we will have a *pandemic* on our hands. A pandemic is an infectious disease that spreads across large distances.

The news is just full of scary things, many of which can make you not want to leave the house. So how is this threat any different than killer bees or the ethnic rainbow of terrorist threats?

Historically, we've had a pandemic influenza every twenty-five to thirty years—roughly the time it takes for the virus to mutate—and we're just about due for the next one. We'd like to think that modern medicine could be our knight in shining armor and that we're done with plagues and pandemics. But a virus is just fighting for survival like the rest of us. To fight each new weapon that comes out of the laboratory, the virus mutates and develops resistance. Having won the battle, it becomes stronger than before.

The other reason we know that this is a real threat is that it has already happened in our recent past. In 1918, we had a pandemic that killed 50 million people worldwide. It began as a bird flu that found a way to spread from person to person. Over half the pregnant women in America died. What is different today from life in 1918 is the impact of modern transportation. What used to take months to travel from country to country can hitchhike around the world in less than a day. Major cities worldwide will be in crisis, with no "outside" help available because there will be no one unaffected outside.

The sky is falling, Chicken Little.
What to do? Run and hide? No, the difference between fear and concern is planning. Local governments are encouraged to have a plan in place for a pandemic. On a very local level, you should have everything you need for at least two to three weeks at your home. Slowly stocking bottled water, vitamins, powdered milk, and canned foods in the pantry is an excellent place to start. Remember not to rush out, stock up, and then forget about it. Buy a little at a time. Monitor the "best before" dates on your stored goods. Use them and replace them on a consistent basis.

Very few of us can afford to stop working and stay home, but we can do our best to minimize our exposure and risks. Every year at flu season it's best to take good care of ourselves; keep unnecessary travel to a minimum and reduce contact with crowds as well. The companies making masks are making a mint, of course, but most of these can offer partial protection at best.

History repeats itself. We can only change how prepared we are and how we come together to survive when it does.

Let Them Play in the Dirt

How do you feel about germs? What about allergens like pet dander and ragweed? These may sound like silly questions, but life is never entirely black and white. According to the hygienic hypothesis, germs and dirt in small doses can actually be your friends.

How is this possible? To start with, our bodies were not made for the sterile environment we've created for ourselves. We were made to play in the dirt and breathe in the ragweed. If someone got sick, they could keep their distance, but they couldn't be isolated from the tribe. We lived without antibacterial wipes and disinfectant sprays, and the more foreign bodies we came in contact with, the stronger we were.

At the center of all this is the way your immune system works. There are two major lines of defense against attack. Your white blood cells are the first line and we're all born with these guys. When an intruder invades, these guys are there to defend. Among this group is a special unit—soldiers with real pre-war intelligence. These specialized white blood cells (called L2) actually build antibodies in advance of an attack. These are the guys that produce an allergic response, which is the direct evidence that they have taken on invaders and beat them before they could do us serious harm.

Your body needs exercise so that your muscles will grow strong and your brain will expand with daily challenges. In the same way, your immune system needs to break a good sweat every now again to stay lean and fighting mean. Without any outside challenges, your first-response white blood cells get lazy. Your immune system needs to practice to stay sharp and keep the delicate balance between these two warriors intact. For people who live protected lives, allergies and autoimmune diseases are more likely to develop. For those who grow up close to nature and rub shoulders with the occasional germ, a healthy life is the more likely outcome.

So what is a parent supposed to do? Sit your kid next to someone with a hacking cough? Tell them to go and play in the mud? The best rule of thumb is moderation in all things. Look out for their best interests, but don't follow them around with antibacterial wipes. Forget about washing hands every time they pet the family dog, but definitely go for the soap and water after the visit to the petting zoo. Let kids be kids. Give them a chance to play in the dirt from time to time. They'll be the envy of their friends.

In your journey to good health, you have to make decisions that sit well with you. If you blindly trust the "experts," you're stuck when they disagree and let down when they change their minds.

When Hospitals Make You Sick

The nightly news is filled with depressing stories of people dying in car accidents and terrible reports of homicides. What we hear very little of is the number of people who suffer and die from hospital-acquired infections. Must be because it's so rare, right?

Wrong. More Americans die each year of hospital-acquired infections than auto accidents and homicides combined. A hospital-acquired infection occurs when someone comes to the hospital with one condition and catches something else. In an age of antibacterial everything, how is this so common? Can we do anything to avoid this? Let's find out.

Hospitals are places where the sick gather, and because of this, wide assortments of germs call the hospital their home. Microscopic armies flourish in catheters and ventilators. Machines and equipment intended to save lives also serve as a locomotive for germs. They can survive for days on hospital rails, bedsheets, and countertops. We have really strong antibacterial cleaners, but they do little good sitting in a box. Even when they are used, they don't always work, thanks to the growing numbers and strains of antibacterial-resistant bacteria (superbugs) out there.

The insurance system is not always set up to help this problem either. They will pay for the extra ten days (average extra stay for those who develop a hospital infection) in the hospital. What they won't pay for is the extra time and staffing necessary to prevent the infection in the first place. Meanwhile, doctors and hospital staff are expected to handle more patients to cut costs.

What can you do to look after your interests if no one else can? There are several things you can do regarding germs. Ask any staff who touches you to wash their hands and equipment. This should include equipment like stethoscopes that go from one bare chest to the next. This may sound a little direct, but you're worth it. You can ask if you can donate your own blood before a surgery in case you need it, to minimize the risk of blood-borne infections. This isn't as extreme as it sounds: there is usually a shortage. Ask if you can go without a catheter or, if the answer is no, request that it be removed at the earliest opportunity. Forty percent of all hospital infections come from the use of urinary catheters, so this would be a big help. Never have body hair shaved right before a surgery if possible. Request to have the hair clipped instead to reduce the risk of infection through abrasions in the skin.

And most important of all, remember that you're in a hospital. This may sound obvious, but with some units of a hospital becoming homier, like maternity wards, folks can let their guard down along with their sanitation levels.

An inherent flaw in our current medical model is the disempowerment created by the hospital and its doctors who hold all the authority and give none to you, the patient. Part of the problem is the term itself. "Patient" implies a sense of helplessness that forces you to sit back and let others control your trip through the hospital system. As the person on the receiving end, your experience is dependent on too many variables that leave you vulnerable. It's better to think of yourself as a partner in your health care. If you have a health crisis or surgery, try to be as educated and informed as you can before you go to the hospital. If you don't know much about the heath field, ask questions and try to have someone with you who can look out after you. If you're not in a position to make coherent decisions, you should have someone with a vested interest in your wellness who can.

Many hospitals are working hard to reduce inherent risks like germs. Some hospitals have cut infection rates nearly in half with the use of a simple checklist before any procedure. A handful of states have passed laws requiring hospitals to report their infection rates. Remember, hospitals are not to be feared. They should be respected for the possibilities they provide and the precautions that are necessary to minimize the risks whenever possible.

Ulcers: A Bacteria Problem

So what causes ulcers? Could it be stress, too much Mexican food, or a spouse who rides you 24/7? Nope, those things can irritate an ulcer you already have, but they're not the root cause.

Our medical knowledge is constantly evolving. What this means is that the conclusions we reach today are often replaced by information that scientists learn tomorrow. This is true with ulcers, too. It is now believed that ulcers can come into being as a result of two possible causes: one is too much medication; the other is a bacterium that goes by the name *H. pylori*.

But wait! What is an ulcer, exactly? Ulcers are open sores that typically appear in the wall of the stomach and/or the small intestines. When the *H. pylori* is the bad guy, an ulcer is an innocent victim of our extremely efficient digestive system.

Think about the way our bodies can take the whole foods we eat and break them down into nutrients, vitamins, proteins, and the like. A lot of that hard work happens in the stomach, where acids and pepsins—strong stuff—go to work on the food and break it apart. What keeps these strong acids from burning a hole though your stomach is a layer of gooey mucus that sticks to the walls and provides a first line of defense. When *H. pylori* sets up camp here, it weakens the mucus and lowers your defenses. Digestive tissue is damaged, and before you know it, you've got an open sore known as an ulcer.

The other reason ulcers occur could be sitting in your medicine cabinet. Drugs called *NSAIDs* are the villains here. These include aspirin, ibuprofen, and allergy meds, among others, that interfere with the body's ability to make an enzyme that produces *prostaglandins*. Prostaglandins are a part of that protective layer we talked about that coats the linings of your stomach and intestine. Their absence can allow harsh digestive juices to damage tissue, causing an ulcer to form.

The pain felt with an ulcer is a burning sensation that can wake you up in the middle of the night when your stomach is empty. You can get lucky and have the pain pass in just a few minutes, or it can hang on for hours. When the ulcer goes deep enough, the inside of your stomach can bleed. You'd notice this blood when vomiting or in bloody stools, which are darker in color.

Okay, we've gone over how ugly this can get. Let's work on getting rid of it. If the ulcer is from your medication, the solution is pretty obvious: change it! If it's an over-the-counter product, look for something more natural to replace it. If it's prescribed, talk to your doctor. In either case, it's a good reason not gobble pills like M&Ms.

If you're not taking these pills, then the problem is bacterial. There are natural cures out there, like *zinc-carnosine*, that really hit the spot. See your natural health-care provider to get started. Oh, one more thing. Just because spicy foods don't cause ulcers doesn't mean you can go out for Mexican tonight. Spicy foods, stress, and six packs will irritate your ulcer big time.

There is always the option to ignore it. But when you do, aren't you ignoring your whole self?

Chapter Four:
Food, Glorious Food

*Life expectancy would grow by leaps and bounds if
green vegetables smelled as good as bacon.*

~Doug Larson

Artificial Sweeteners: A not so Sweet Deal

To tell the story of artificial sweeteners, we have to go all the way back to
1879 at Johns Hopkins University. There, two chemists were diligently
working at making new chemical dyes from tar derivatives when one
of their concoctions boiled over and spilled onto one scientist's hands.
At his next meal (after no hand washings), he noticed how sweet his
fingers tasted, and saccharin, our first artificial sweetener, was born.
Since then, many more have sprung up. Although they carry the
FDA's seal of approval, many think they should get booted out of the
food chain.

There are many sweeteners out there because different chemicals
behave differently. Splenda can withstand heat, so it's used in baking
goods; sugar alcohols do not affect blood sugar, so it's the sugar
substitute marketed to diabetics. You can also find sweeteners in sweet
products that shouldn't use sugar, like most toothpaste and even some
conventional vitamins. Aspartame is much cheaper than sugar, so it has
been added to nondiet products, all in the name of economics.

So how does something with so few calories give me such sweet ice
cream and soda? It's much sweeter than sugar, so only a tiny drop is

needed. Saccharin packs a punch 300 times sweeter than its natural counterpart!

As statistics show that we are not getting any smaller, the natural assumption is that a few diet chemicals are a better alternative to adding a notch on our belts. Eating foods with no calories should translate into a smaller you, right? Not according to a recent Purdue study, where it was learned that when people eat artificially sweetened food, the body loses its ability to "keep track" of calories. The natural link between sweetness and calories is lost; our bodies miscalculate when we eat real sugar, and we end up weighing more.

So where is the health controversy? Is the FDA sleeping on the job? Each sweetener has its own story to tell, but we'll go over saccharin today because it has one of the seediest pasts. In 1977, the FDA tried but failed to ban it due to animal studies, which showed its link to cancer. It didn't get pulled from the shelves, even though foods containing saccharin did carry a warning label until the 1990s. In 2000, Congress removed it from the list of cancer-causing substances, and it's now called safe by the FDA. Meanwhile, there are many groups that link this sticky sweet stuff to everything from headaches to Alzheimer's disease, making the issue a muddy one indeed.

What is clear is that at some level, you have to know this stuff is a trick and your body doesn't like being fooled. And at the end of the day, the laugh comes at the high price of your health. So the next time you love your food, ask if this food is nurturing and loving you back.

Why We Should "Can" the Bottled Water

"Oh man, I've given up those nasty sodas and sugary fruit drinks. Now they're picking on water. Are we getting just a little too picky?" It's true that, hands down, water is your best bet when it comes to hydrating your body and that, for years, being seen around town with bottled water was a status symbol for the healthy. But when it comes to the exotic brands that have emerged in recent years, would Mother Nature approve?

Living in the middle of a bustling city, one can see the appeal of bottled water with names like Alaska Water or Glacier Clear. You can almost picture those guys in their snowsuits hiking to that crystal-pure, half-frozen stream to bottle your water. The problem is that most bottled water is not captured from such pristine places. The Alaska water that comes from Alaska is from the municipal water in Juneau; Glacier Clear bottles their water in Greenville, Tennessee. Many of these "health conscious" companies make soda, too. Aquafina is made by PepsiCo, and the folks at Coca-Cola give us Dasani. The FDA actually admits to being more lax on bottled water than the stuff that comes from our tap.

There is also the question of leaching. While the jury is still out among academics, most of us believe there is something not quite right when it comes to the plastic bottles. Why? Some plastics have PVCs added to make them more flexible. When this concoction is heated, chemicals from the bottle can leach into the water.

When the water is gone, the bottles remain. The bottled water industry uses about 2.7 million tons of plastic each year to make those bottles. Roughly 10 percent make it to the recycling bin. The rest take about a thousand years to degrade, and when they do, it's not pretty. It's scary to think that the use of bottled water is contributing to our need for it. Some of these bottles are world travelers. Fiji water bottles are transported all the way from China. Can you smell the oil fumes?

In the end, your health gets bruised from bottled water while Mother Earth gets TKO'd. It's better to stick to the tap and get a filter for peace of mind. You can even try reverse osmosis or distilling if you're up for it. When you're on the go, try a bottle you can reuse, like one made of stainless steel.

Think of your health as a work in progress. I've often heard you can only do best for what you know at the time. And now that you know, it's time to "can" the bottle.

Fats: The Good, the Bad, and the Ugly

Fat is bad. Fat is bad.

If you've been dieting, this may be your mantra when it comes to fats. While it's true that most of us get more than our share of fat, we actually need a certain amount of fat in our diets. Why? Two great reasons are these: some of our vitamins are stored in fat for safekeeping, and our cells are lined with fats.

The challenge is that all fats are not created equally. Some are bad, some are good, some are absolutely essential for our well-being, and others are just toxic. The trick is to choose the right kind of fats to help your body run better.

First we'll start with the good type: *omega 3*. Omega 3 fatty acids are mostly found in freshwater fish, such as salmon. You can also find smaller amounts in flaxseeds and walnuts. Omega 3 fatty acids are essential for good health and proper brain function. They help protect against heart disease and cancer. In fact, omega 3 fatty acids are at the top of the who's who list when it comes to good health. If you only plan to do one good thing for your health, this would be it. Don't like fish? Not to worry, just get a good omega 3 supplement.

Monounsaturated and *polyunsaturated* fats also live on the good side of the pendulum. These fats are liquid at room temperature. These are the vegetable oils, peanut oils, avocados, and most nuts. Fats coming from animals are *saturated* fats and fall into the bad category. These fats are solid or waxy at room temperature. Not to say you should never eat a good, locally grown, juicy burger every once in a while or nice piece of lamb, but they should be consumed in moderation.

Now, on to the ugly. The next fat explains why your Twinkie will never go bad. Why, when you buy a candy bar or processed peanut butter you don't have to look at the expiration date, because that date is a time far, far away, in a distant galaxy. *Trans-fatty acids* are fats created in a lab and are in a lot of the processed foods you buy. An extra hydrogen molecule is added on the fat to increase the shelf life of the food, not the life of the person consuming it. The current debate over this fat isn't whether this fat is good or bad for you, but rather how bad is it, exactly. No kidding! If the conversation goes something like, "Is it just kind of toxic or a proven cancer-causing killer?" then the answer should be to steer clear of it. How do you recognize it? Just look for "trans-fats" or "partially hydrogenated oil" hiding in the list of ingredients.

Your body is your temple. You want to build it using nothing but the finest materials.

Gluten Intolerance: So Long, Bottom of the Food Pyramid

We all remember the food pyramid. It's the American guide to what to eat. But just as we change our living quarters to reflect our changing needs, it's time to take a look at the cramped quarters we've assigned to fruits and veggies and consider moving them to the spacious accommodations currently enjoyed by breads and cereals.

In spite of consistent increases in obesity and diabetes in our population, breads and cereals continue to get the lion's share of the recommended daily diet. Though our government agencies have been slow to respond and manufacturers continue to produce and promote processed foods, our bodies are sending clear messages that things have got to change. For many of us, these foods are increasingly off limits as our systems no longer tolerate them.

Gluten intolerance is one condition that is often poorly understood and in many cases goes misdiagnosed. We're not talking allergies here: this is intolerance. Much of the good stuff your body takes from food happens in the intestines. The inside of your intestines are like a '70s shag carpet, full of projections called *villi*. These little tentacles pluck out nutrients and water as they roll by. For someone who is gluten intolerant, eating a bagel will cause the intestines to wear down its thick shag carpet until it looks like cheap vinyl flooring. Without the villi, the body can't absorb nutrients. Instead of feeding its needs, it just sends it out the other end.

What does intolerance look like? It often goes misdiagnosed because the symptoms are not unique. Gas, bloating, diarrhea, and abdominal pain are some of the digestive ones. Other symptoms, such as joint pain, muscle cramps, mouth sores, and menstrual cramps, are easily mistaken for something else. Left untreated, it can lead to malnutrition. In infants, it can lead to failure to thrive. Your chances of getting cancer go up, too, if you're gluten intolerant and fail to follow a gluten-free diet.

It seems crazy that our bodies would reject a natural food group. What possible reason would my body have for rejecting a beautiful blueberry muffin, for instance? What about a slice of freshly baked whole-grain bread? How can that be bad for me?

As always, the body has a reason, and in this case, we have to look to our past. Centuries ago, our hairier ancestors did not have bakeries right down the street. Grains were an infrequent addition to our diet, unlike today, when breads and pasta figure so prominently. For a species whose digestive system is more naturally geared to veggies, meat, and fruit, grains are uninvited guests. One could take it a step further and say that those who are gluten intolerant have smarter bodies that simply won't put up with processed fluff.

What is great news is that once you take all gluten out of your diet, the symptoms start to go away. What is a challenge is figuring out how to avoid gluten. First, you need to stay away from all wheat, barley or rye … and that's the easy part. Many food additives, such as malt flavoring, contain gluten. You can't stop there either. Your vitamins and medications need to be scrutinized, too; and if you cohabit with a bread-eater, watch out for her crumbs getting into your peanut butter jar; make sure that your sweetie doesn't make your eggs in the pan used to make pancakes.

Eating out is a challenge, which means you'll end up eating most of your meals at home. It may be hard to leave behind the foods we love, but if we listen to our bodies, it will be much easier for them to love us back.

Honey: A Natural Healer?

Ancient Olympians ate honey to improve their athletic performance. Egyptian goddesses put honey on their faces for beautiful skin. Hippocrates used it to heal sores and ulcers on his patients. Even in the "modern" world, honey is favored by opera singers for its unique abilities to heal the throat. For most of us, though, honey is just something we occasionally slap on our toast. Does it deserve more respect? Let's take a closer look at bees' gold and find out why it's more than a sugar substitute.

Next time you get a minor cut or burn, try slapping a little natural honey on it. In a study out of India involving 104 first-degree burn patients, 91 percent treated with honey were infection free compared to 7 percent receiving conventional treatment. What's more, the honey-treated group healed faster!

What's the science behind this, you wonder? Honey is composed of both glucose and fructose. These are two sugars that strongly attract water. In other words, the honey pulls water from the wound, drying it up so that moisture-loving bacteria and fungi are kept at bay. To sweeten the deal even further, honey in its raw form also has antimicrobial agents to keep infection away.

Honey naturally has antioxidants, too. These can pick up free radicals in the body and move them out of your system. Free radicals are the seeds of cancer, so you want as few of these as possible. We all have free radicals floating around in our systems, and honey consumed daily will help lower that population.

Not all honey is created equal. The quality of the honey is only as healthful as the plants the bees feed on. Consuming local honey is best, because it can help protect us from local allergens. Heating honey will burn off many of its natural healing properties, so it's best to keep it cool. The darker the honey, the more rich it is in antioxidants. Raw honey is best, which can usually be hunted down in places like farmers' markets.

Honey offers incredible benefits for diabetics and those with high cholesterol, and we never even mentioned how great it tastes! Natural raw honey deserves a prominent place in your kitchen and your medicine cabinet because it works so many wonders as a healing agent and a delicious food ... with one exception: honey is *not* a food for babies. Botulism occurs naturally in our environment and naturally in honey. At less than twelve months of age, a baby's digestive system has not yet matured, which means that a baby can easily develop botulism from honey.

Got Lactose Intolerance?

Got gas? Got bloating? Got a crampy feeling in your tummy after a glass of milk or slice of cheese pizza? You may have *lactose intolerance*. Lactose intolerance is the inability to properly digest the sugar (lactose) found in milk. All of that gas and bloating is your body's way of saying, "I can't break this down into energy."

Millions of Americans have lactose intolerance and don't even know it. Almost all of us are born with plenty of *lactase*, enough to live on our mom's beautiful milk for months without any troubles. Lactase is what our bodies produce to help us digest milk sugar or lactose. As we get older, our lactase level naturally goes down, and for two-thirds of the world's population, our ability to digest lactose plummets to a level where we're considered intolerant. These levels vary by ethnic origin. Only about 15 percent of people of northern European descent are intolerant compared to numbers as high as 95 percent for people of Asian and African descent.

Could you be lactose intolerant and not even know it? A sure sign is a gassy, bloated feeling after a meal, which is definitely not a normal digestive phase. Some people who are highly lactose intolerant get misdiagnosed with irritable bowel syndrome and have no idea that the answer to their problem could be as simple as changing the milk products in their diet.

You can get tested for lactose intolerance in a medical office or start your own investigation by drinking two tall glasses of milk and waiting to see the result. Most symptoms occur half an hour to two hours after, as your body tries to digest the lactose. You could also try going a week without dairy and see how you feel.

Remember that we're not talking about an allergy here; an allergy involves a reaction of your immune system. This is a question of digestion. Some people with lactose intolerance can handle some dairy, while others can clear a room after a slice of cheese pizza.

If you discover that your body has trouble with dairy, fret not. You don't have to give up ice cream or anything else you've come to love because there are plenty of healthy substitutions that don't contain milk. Fill your cereal bowl with rice milk; have some almond nut ice cream on a hot afternoon. Your favorite health food store is packed with tasty alternate choices, and your body still needs its daily servings of calcium. So eat plenty of dark veggies, almonds, soymilk, and oranges, all of which naturally contain calcium. Take a good calcium supplement for added insurance so that your bones will be strong for years to come.

With just a few simple changes and modifications, lactose intolerance can be easily managed.

Eating Organic

You're in the grocery store. In one hand you hold a conventional apple; in the other you hold one whose sticker lets you know that it was organically grown. You know the organic one is a little pricier, but organic foods sound better, and you've heard good things about them. What to do?

Let's start by defining "organic" before we go into why it's good for us. There are four basic categories when it comes to organic. First, there is "100 percent organic." Foods bearing this label should be the real deal—all organic. Next, there is "FDA certified organic"; only 95 percent of the ingredients need be organic here. The next level down is "made with organic"; this requires 70 percent organic ingredients. Anything less than 70 percent means that a manufacturer can only list the organic items in the ingredients.

Most folks who pay a little extra for organic aren't just paying for the extras they're getting; they're paying for what they're not getting, too. These "extras" include the chemicals, hormones, and pesticides that are added to the regular foods. People who buy organic apples just want the apple and nothing more.

One reason organic produce is more expensive is the added work organic farmers have to do. They cannot use sewage sludge, genetically modified organisms, irradiation (which is done at the same wavelength as an X-ray), or growth hormones. If a farmer wants to switch his land over to organic, a three-year waiting period is required to ensure the land is pesticide free.

Let's move on to the nutrition debate and look at the question, is organic food better for you? Researchers are still hard at work, meaning that the jury has yet to decide that organic is a clear winner. Many large growers are reluctant to climb aboard the organic train, given the costs, so there is some resistance there.

What has been found without question is that the soil in organic farms contains much higher levels of antioxidants, vitamins, and minerals, meaning that these higher concentrations find their way into the organic produce they sustain.

Organic food doesn't have all the extra pesticides and additives that come from a chemistry lab. Livestock on organic farms need to have an outdoor area for the animals to roam (not required for nonorganic farmers). The animals breathe fresh air, not stale air filled with the airborne pollutants living in barns, coops, and pens. Going organic isn't just for those who dine on seaweed chips and tofu bars. Almost everything you can imagine is available in organic form, from meats to fruits and vegetables, to coffee to potato chips. You name it ... it's your food, only better.

So there you have it. Make yourself a priority. You're worth it.

Organic Whole Foods: The Apple in Your Apple Pie

Yum, I just love organic apples. Organic bananas: those are good, too. Without all those nasty pesticides and assorted chemical, time-altering enhancements, I can eat anything so long as it's organic, right? Organic pizza, organic power bars, cheese crackers shaped like cute little bunnies ... What could we have against cute little bunnies?

Don't get me wrong: I like my food as chemical free as the next person, but organic isn't a license to eat processed sweets, which means that a good part of what we eat should be both organic and whole. So let's discuss why a lemon is sometimes better than lemonade.

This might seem a bit basic to some, but the first thing we should do is define "whole foods." Whole foods are things you find naturally produced by Mother Nature without help from us: fruits, vegetables, and whole grains like brown rice and cornmeal; beans, nuts, and seeds; eggs, seafood, and fowl. These foods come with no ingredient list.

Foods that are good for you are also the ones that go bad after sitting in your pantry for too long. The concept is pretty simple. We are a part of the earth. It makes sense that we benefit most from products of this beautiful blue ball we sit on.

Let's take the tuna as an example. By now, most of us know about omega 3 fatty acids: the good cancer-fighting, healthy fat. Fresh from the boat, most whole, cooked tuna packs about 3 grams of omega 3s per serving. Take that same amount of tuna out of a can, and you get half the omega 3 value with a whole lot more unhealthy fat. Why? Most canned tuna is found swimming in inferior vegetable oil. And these are just the nutrients that we know about. We are always "discovering" something that has been quietly sitting in whole foods for years.

So, hands down, the organic chocolate bar beats its conventional counterpart. But let's not forget that it's still a chocolate bar that belongs in the category marked "other."

Put a priority on fresh fruits, veggies, and nuts in your diet. Trust Mother Nature. Her formula has worked so much longer than ours.

Soft Drinks: The Hard Truth

Imagine you grew up on a remote island eating what you could fish, find, or gather. You'd fill your belly with nutrients and be in great shape. Now imagine a plane dropped a six-pack of soda. Do you think your body would like this fizzy drink? Would you wonder if it was really food?

Soda accounts for more than a quarter of all drinks consumed in the United States, despite the fact that almost everyone knows that they're bad for us. Ever wonder why we keep drinking this stuff?

If we're going to talk soda, we need to talk sugar. We all know that each little can is chocked full of sugar, but just how much? Brace yourselves: on average, one can of soda packs ten teaspoons of sugar! In fact, soft drink manufacturers are the largest single user of refined sugar in this big beautiful country.

When we think of sugar, we might first think how it shows up on the bathroom scale. Then we might think about the holes or cavities it causes in our teeth. Then there's the insulin spike in our blood. With enough sugar, your pancreas eventually throws up a white surrender flag and type-2 diabetes becomes a reality. Do you think this is extreme? Studies show that 21 percent of those over sixty in the United States have diabetes, with these numbers on the rise.

We've all heard the term "empty calories" before, but what does it mean for your body? Our body gets us out and about every day. To do this, it has a grocery list of nutrients it needs to keep everything running smoothly. Let's take vitamin C for example. Vitamin C performs over 300 tasks, including helping those germ-fighting white blood cells of ours. Two kiwis and an orange would stack up just right for the ideal daily serving (about 250 mg) and contribute 150 calories.

Okay, to maintain our ideal weight we need to consume 1,600 to 2,400 calories a day. Let's say you're a short-ish female with a 1,600-a-day calorie intake. Your vitamin C intake leaves you with lots of room for other good things. If you chose a sixty-four-ounce Big Gulp soda instead, you just consumed 800 calories and your body received no nutrition whatsoever. By the way, this is how we end up with a population that is both malnourished and overweight.

And would you care to take a guess what soda does for your bones? One ingredient in most popular colas is phosphoric acid. Too much of this acid promotes the loss of calcium throughout your skeleton, leaving your bones weak and porous and more likely to fracture.

Let's look at the balance sheet. With soda, diet or not, we add nothing good to support and nurture our bodies while we fill up on empty, processed calories. We litter the planet with bottles and cans and spend our hard-earned dollars on consumables that quickly fizzle out and leave us both fat and flat. No matter how much you may love the taste of soda, it will never love or nourish you back.

Before you buy your next fizzy treat, ask yourself this ... When your body wears out, where will you live?

Does Sugar Act Alone in the Harvesting of Cavities

Ohhh, the sound of a dentist's drill. Not many noises can make your hair stand on end quite like that. But the pain you're going through is all your fault. You had plenty of time to indulge in too many powdered doughnuts but not enough time to use the free dental floss your dentist gave you on your last visit.

Yes, it's true we gobble down sugar in this country just like candy. And it's also true that not enough of our time in front of the mirror is spent grooming our teeth. But there's more to the softening of our teeth than sweets and laziness can account for, so let's brush up on the reasons we get cavities.

Do you know someone who can nibble on sweets all day long and when it's their turn to go for their cleaning, they come home with a perfect report card and never need any follow-up visits?

Do you know others who seem to get cavities just thinking about sweets, no matter how much they scrub and floss their teeth?

The answer to this mystery is bacteria, which loves plaque, that whitish, sticky stuff that hangs out near the gum line. The ingredients in plaque block the saliva from rinsing the tooth enamel where they're located. In this plaque ecosphere, the bacteria feed. As a by-product, bacteria release acid that eats away at your teeth and causes cavities.

Each of us supports different populations of bacteria, which means that some of us have a tougher challenge keeping our teeth whole. To win the battle, if not the war, we should be brushing out teeth with a gentle brush for two to three minutes at a time. Most of us shave this ritual down to a measly thirty seconds. As for flossing, my favorite slogan comes from a former dentist of mine. He had a sign in his office that read, "You don't have to floss all your teeth … just the ones you want to keep."

Since sugars and simple starches do so little good for our bodies, it doesn't hurt us at all to stay away from them. Our teeth are just the first insult sugar slings at us on its free ride through our digestive system. Stick to fruit in its natural state and drink plenty of water. After that, talk to your dentist. He or she is the real expert on how best to maintain your oral health.

In health, what matters most is how we manage the hand we are dealt.

SECTION TWO:
HOW WE COPE ... AND DON'T!

The ... patient should be made to understand that he
or she must take charge of his own life. Don't take your
body to the doctor as if he were a repair shop.

~ Quentin Regestein

When you consider all the stresses and strains we put ourselves through, it's pretty incredible that our bodies keep on keeping on as well as they do.

What is even more amazing is how well protected we are by our body's defenses. We often forget that our personal army is always on duty, even when we're asleep.

This section takes a look at the many ways that we enjoy its protections, at the warning signals it sends us when we're under attack, and the rare occasions when it tells us that it's had enough.

- Chapter 1 outlines the reactions we experience
- Chapter 2 explains causes and symptoms associated with conditions and syndromes
- Chapter 3 describes several familiar behaviors
- Chapter 4 takes a look at diseases
- Chapter 5 gives an overview of some common viruses and allergies
- Chapter 6 brings us a better understanding of the effects of pregnancy
- Chapter 7 alerts us to the power controlled by our hormones

Chapter One:
Reactions

The appearance of a disease is swift as an arrow;
its disappearance slow, like a thread.

~ Chinese Proverb

When the Bee Stings

It's a beautiful day. You're out in your garden. The veggies are almost ready for your plate, and the fruit is ripe. You feel at one with nature. Just when you think everything is perfect, someone who had been dining on your pretty flowers has mistaken you as enemy number one and now you've been stung.

Bee stings are no one's idea a good time, so let's swarm over some ideas of how to handle them.

Once the stinger is lodged into your skin, you may be tempted to pinch it out of there, but that's not such a good idea. The bee's stinger actually has a venom sac inside it, and pinching it will squeeze more of the poison into your body. Using a straight-edged object to scrape it off is best. Some recommend a credit card or the dull side of a knife to do the trick. Even if your fingernails are short, they're probably long enough to scrape the stinger out and that way you don't have to waste any time looking around.

The next thing you want to do is get some ice on it to control the swelling. If you're a frequent victim of bee stings, you will swell up even more. The swelling is the body's way of flushing out the venom, but it can sometimes get a little carried away. You should keep applying ice for twenty minutes at a time until the swelling goes down.

Now let's look at some home remedies. Meat tenderizers work really well. Mix with water so it becomes a paste and apply directly to your skin. A bee's venom is protein based, and meat tenderizer breaks down the protein. (It also works well on jellyfish stings, by the way.) Relief should come in a matter of sixty seconds or less.

If you're a vegetarian, you probably don't have meat tenderizer on hand. An alternative option is baking soda mixed with water and made into a paste. Apply it directly to your skin. This works almost as well, but the tenderizer takes first place.

For more serious situations, you need to get professional help. If you have any difficulty breathing or you feel dizzy, this is a medical emergency. You need to get on the phone and call for an ambulance. Some people's bodies overreact to a sting and their reaction can escalate fast. In a case like this, be thankful for the outside help.

To prevent future attacks, avoid wearing bright colors. If you plan to spend the day outside, know that your fruity perfume beckons unwanted bees to your side. Never swat at bees, as they will take that action as hostile and go on the attack.

When you do get stung, don't think poorly of the bee. They do give us honey, a yummy and healthful food. Remember that for you it's just a sting: for the bee, it's a kamikaze mission.

Sun Damage … a Major Burn

Summertime: festivals and outdoor activities abound. After a long winter, it's time to pull out the T-shirts and tank tops and go for that beautiful bronzed look. You know—the one that makes you look a size smaller and your teeth a shade whiter.

Which means that it's also time to start growing roughed skin, red veins on your cheeks, and wrinkles that would put Old Mother Hubbard to shame because that "natural glow" has a dark ugly side. While skin cancer is by far the most devastating effect of too much ultraviolet radiation, let's not make fear our theme. Instead, let's appeal to our vanity for reasons to skip the sun baking.

We'll begin by looking for the first sign of sun damage. A suntan is an injury to the top layer of your skin. While the sun beams down on your skin, your body puts up a defense, pulling down the shade by mass-producing melanin to block the UV rays. All this extra melanin gives you a tan, which means that your "natural glow" is your body trying to defend itself.

The signature of sunburn is red skin. It's red because the cells of your skin are inflamed. The swelling is caused when your body brings blood to the surface to repair the burned skin cells. Soaps, perfumes, and other chemicals can heighten the effects of the burn. The skin can become tight, and the lightest touch brushing up against it can bring tears.

What does a lifetime of tanning and burning get you? In the beginning, overtanned cells will be permanently darkened, giving you freckles. UV rays can make the skin paper thin, painting your face and body with fine lines and wrinkles. This also opens the door to tears and cuts in your skin. Thin skin also has trouble holding water, so it dries out pretty fast, meaning deeper lines and wrinkles. Many sessions of inflammation can cause the elastin in your skin to get tangled up. When this happens, it's called *elastosis*. It can be spotted as yellow thickened bumps on the skin. After every burn, the capillaries in your skin become congested and don't always spring back into shape. They can stamp your skin in the form of dilated red vessels or red cherry spots, most often found on the face. And don't forget those large brown lesions, which go by the attractive name of liver spots.

So what is the bottom line? Buy a big sunhat and leave the leather skin for the cows. Slap on some chemical-free sunscreen. Know that radiation is something that adds up over a lifetime. Even if you are young and invincible, you need to start caring for yourself now. We do need the healing effects of the sun, but only for about twenty minutes a day, without the baby oil. Your skin is the biggest organ in the body. Protect your birthday suit. It looks great in the color you got it in.

You Give Me Fever

What do you do when you get a fever? Do you automatically reach into the medicine cabinet? Do you try to track down the culprit who selfishly shared this illness with you? What may surprise you is that a fever is actually your body's way of fighting off a virus or bacteria. The fever itself is not a disease but a sign that your body is doing its best to defend you. In fact, your body is so smart that it will raise your temperature just high enough to weaken the particular virus or bacteria it's trying to wipe out.

This means that there are actually times when taking over-the-counter meds like Tylenol or aspirin to bring the fever down may actually work against your body's good intentions and prolong the illness. They don't give the body a chance to fight the disease naturally, a process that makes the immune system stronger for the battles yet to come. Not only that, but both of these pain medications have side effects; too much aspirin can irritate the stomach lining and can cause bleeding ulcers, while Tylenol taken in frequent doses can affect the liver adversely.

Normal body temperature ranges from 97 to 99 degrees Fahrenheit, varying throughout the day. Usually it's lower in the morning and higher in the late afternoon. Any temperature above 100 degrees is considered to be a fever.

During a fever, drink plenty of liquids to avoid dehydration. Bathe frequently. Bathing helps in two ways. A lukewarm bath can help bring down a temperature naturally if it's getting too high (over 102 degrees). Regular bathing can also help wash away toxins that your body releases through the skin. During a fever you sweat more and there are more toxins to be released. Allowing these substances to stay on your skin can present the opportunity for them to be reabsorbed.

Although a fever is usually a natural self-defense mechanism, this does not mean that it should be ignored. Your body needs rest so that it can take care of itself.

You also need to be mindful of any symptoms that are trying to tell you if this is more than an ordinary fever. Check with your health-care provider if the fever lasts longer than three days or reaches 103 degrees or more.

A severe headache or neck stiffness with a fever can be a sign of something more serious, and medical attention should be sought right away. Be extra vigilant with the very young, with seniors, and with those who have preexisting conditions.

Remember, a fever is a symptom that your body is working hard to maintain balance. The next time you get a fever, don't feel cheated by your body. Think of it as a cleansing process that is getting rid of toxins and infections.

I Got a Headache This Big

All things are not created equal, as we know, and this is true of headaches, too. In general, headaches are classified into two groups: vascular and nonvascular. *Vascular* headaches include cluster headaches, hypertension headaches, and the dreaded migraine. *Nonvascular* headaches, or those not caused by blood vessels, are called tension headaches; they are usually caused by tight muscles in the neck.

Tension Headaches

The feeling that a vise grip has been applied to the skull is a pretty common description of a tension headache. It often starts at the back of the skull and spreads over the entire head. When it gets really bad, people can feel the pain at the back of their eyes. There is no throbbing or pounding, as with migraines; this pain is a constant, dull ache.

The easiest way to diagnose a tension headache is by applying pressure to your neck muscles. If this worsens or relieves the pain, you have a tension headache.

On rare occasions, a jaw being out of place may cause a tension headache. Most of the time, however, a tension headache is caused by the tightening in the muscles of the face, neck, or scalp as a result of stress and/or poor posture. The tightening of the muscle results in the pinching of a nerve or its blood supply; this, in turn, results in the sensation of pain and pressure.

What to do? If you get tension headaches, a good first step is learning how to relax. When we get stressed out, some of us bite our nails, some of us reach for a favorite snack, and a lot of us tense the muscles in our necks. Next time you're feeling stressed, look in the mirror and see if your shoulders are trying to reach your earlobes. If this sounds like you, try exhausting your shoulder muscles by tensing them and holding them that way for thirty seconds. When you relax your shoulders again, they should feel like they hang lower.

When a misalignment in the spine creates muscular tension in the neck, chiropractic care can be quite helpful. In fact, tension headaches respond very well to bodywork in general. Becoming aware of your body posture and tension levels is necessary for long-term change. Whatever you do, remember that a tension headache is not something that you have to learn to live with. It's a condition that you can prevent!

"One pill makes you larger and one pill makes you small;
And the ones that mother gives you don't do anything at all."

The Misunderstood Migraine

These lyrics come to us from Grace Slick in her interpretation of *Alice, Through the Looking Glass*. Written by Lewis Carroll more than a century ago, Alice's adventures were inspired in part by Carroll's personal experience as a migraine sufferer whose search for a cure led him to try many medications that altered his perceptions of the world in strange and wondrous ways.

Millions of Americans suffer from migraines each year, yet they remain one of the least understood and most widely misdiagnosed diseases out there. Migraines get dismissed as "bad" headaches all the time, usually by those who have never experienced them firsthand. In fact, there is an enormous difference that goes far beyond the degree of severity.

A headache is a symptom—a sign the body is sending that something is wrong. The sufferer could be dehydrated, stressed out and tense, or they could simply have hit their head. The end result is that not enough blood gets to the brain.

A migraine is a disease caused by *vasodilation*—a condition in which the vessels that carry blood around your body grow bigger in diameter—leading to the delivery of too much blood to the brain. Since most headache medication is designed to *increase* blood flow, migraine sufferers should never take regular headache medication; doing so can actually make the pain worse.

How do you tell if you are suffering from migraines? In the first place, migraines are genetically based, meaning that you probably have a blood relative who suffers from them, too.

Migraine symptoms include a throbbing pain on one side of the head. All of your senses are heightened: light seems brighter, colors are more intense, noises are louder, the chemicals in food are more noticeable, and the sense of touch is more acute, including the atmospheric pressure on your body.

A migraine is often triggered by menstrual cycles, thanks to the drop in estrogen levels; bright lights; aspartame sweetener; alcohol; and weather conditions. In Germany, for example, there is a hotline that migraine sufferers call to find out if the day's forecasted weather is likely to trigger a migraine.

At this time there is no cure for migraines. The best that sufferers can do is to avoid their triggers and manage the symptoms. To add insult to injury, sufferers also have to put up with society's misunderstanding of the disorder. Sufferers are frequently dismissed as chronic complainers who can't handle normal levels of stress and often have difficulty getting time off when an episode occurs. So, the next time you meet someone with a migraine, don't offer unhelpful suggestions to cheer up and/or grow up. Try to be a part of their solution and help them find a quiet, dimly lit place to rest until the episode has passed.

What Makes Your Knuckles Crack and Pop?

Folks often walk into my office and ask about a shoulder, hip, or knuckles they can pop. Some are just curious while others wonder if their knuckles could swell up and swallow their rings. Can cracking your knuckles or any other joint cause arthritis? Is this just an old wives' tale? And what causes that loud "take no prisoners" noise anyway? Let's find out.

What's behind a *cavitation*? The spaces between the bones in your body are your joints. These joints are laced together by rope-like ligaments. To keep your bones moving smoothly, a clear liquid called *synovial fluid* is encased in each joint. When you contort your fingers to make them crack, you are pulling apart your bones. This increases the area for your joint fluid to swim in. As with any liquid, an increase in space brings about a decrease in pressure. This drop in pressure turns liquid into a gas, and tiny bubbles form. Eventually, the pressure builds up, and just like bubble wrap, they give off a loud pop. Ever wonder why it takes about half an hour to repeat the offence? That's about the time it takes your body to absorb those tiny bubbles.

So, is cracking your knuckles bad for you? Well there's not a ton of research out there (can you believe they have bigger fish to fry), but so far no link has been found between cracking and arthritis. What has been discovered is a different kind of damage. In a study conducted with 300 knuckle-crackers, soft-tissue damage to the joint capsule and ligaments was found, along with a decrease in grip strength. Over time, all that popping and pulling simply wears you down.

"But why does it feel good?" When you crack any joint in your body, a set of nerve endings called *Golgi tendon organs* are stimulated. Your body responds by relaxing the muscles around that joint. The fact that we feel good after a good crack doesn't mean that it's good for us, so the next time you feel the urge to crack your knuckles, try rubbing them instead.

Motion Sickness: A Choppy Ride

Ahhh, another beautiful day and another beautiful reason to head out on the open road. Maybe your destination is a sheltered picnic spot, a historic ruin, or the mesmerizing rhythmic beat of the ocean breaking on your favorite beach.

If you're one of those who, while looking at the beautiful roadside view, are also looking for possible places to pull over, motion sickness is a terrible way to ruin your day. If your case is really extreme, a winding road sign might as well be a road closed sign. To give comfort and ensure smooth sailing ahead, let's try to navigate a path through the choppy world of motion sickness.

Motion sickness brings with it a feeling of uneasiness, a cold sweat, and that sudden upheaval for a grand finale. The young and the elderly are especially vulnerable, but anyone can fall victim.

Motion sickness is a disagreement between different motion sensors in the body. We have several ways to detect motion and determine our relative position. How does our body tell us if we're lying down or standing? Our eyes send signals to the brain to let us know where we are; in the dark, we rely on sensory nerves telling us if there's pressure on our feet or across our body; and our middle ear detects position and movement. Usually they work together to give us a complete picture of our position. Motion sickness is when they disagree. So when you're sitting in a moving vehicle, reading, your eyes and sensory nerves think you're sitting still while your inner ear thinks your body is doing gymnastics. The argument they have gives you that uneasy, queasy sensation that doesn't go away until everything has had a chance to settle down, after the motion has stopped.

Some of us never go on the spine-tingling rides at a theme park without needing a barf bag; others handle upside-down-inside-out rides without batting an eyelash. The key to handling motion sickness is prevention. After the pale green monster has arrived, nothing can stop it. But there are some ways to keep your body in agreement. In a plane, try reserving a seat by the wings, the steadiest section on an aircraft. On a boat, the cabin nearest the center of the ship moves the least, so book that and plan to spend plenty of time on deck, looking at the horizon. Take ginger tablets to keep the stomach calm. Ginger (or in a pinch, ginger ale) helps prevent the nausea and queasiness of motion sickness.

If motion sickness sickens you, you can sit back and wonder why me or take steps to help your body adjust to a world that sometimes leave everyone a little confused.

What a Pain in the Neck: "Hold Your Head High"

For most people, this is a reminder to be confident and proud. In my line of work, I like to take a more literal interpretation: not to slouch and to take care of your neck.

But what happens when your neck isn't being cared for the way it cares for you? Poor posture, arthritis, and accidents can all lead to neck pain. Because your neck is much more than a place your noggin sits upon, let's look at the area between your head and shoulders and find out what can happen when it doesn't get the care and attention it deserves.

Let's start with a little light anatomy. In order to get the range of motion necks have, a little bit of stability had to be sacrificed. Your neck has seven bones stacked up on top of one another. In between those bones are disks, which are cushiony pillows that keep the bones from grinding against each other when you turn you head. Ligaments are the ropes that lock these bones together. Then there are the muscles, which use tendons to grab hold of the bones. The muscles are the movers and shakers at this party. Finally, there are the nerves that use the spine as their freeway to get messages to and from the brain.

"So why does my neck hurt?" It's a question I get many times a day. Any combination of the parts listed above can be a source of your pain in the neck. Your bones can whittle down with age, and arthritis can set in. This is seven times more likely if you've ever had whiplash, by the way. The hardworking muscles in your neck can become strained. This is where posture can really play a role. In profile, your ears should sit directly above your shoulders. If your head juts forward a few inches, you're overworking the muscles in the back of your neck.

Try this simple test to see if your posture is working against you. Find an empty wall in your house and back up to it. Your head and back should hit at the same time. If not, you're carrying your head too far forward!

Your disks can also wear down, causing the bones to be too close for comfort. This squeeze can cause the three-lane highway your nerves travel in to get in a pinch and become just a single-lane construction zone.

Adding one last piece to the puzzle is the fact that neck pain is not always a "point to where it hurts" situation. Tight muscles in the back of the neck can cause a headache, shoulder pain, or create a pins-and-needles sensation that can run right down to your fingers. Conversely, you can have something out of place from the jaw, head, or shoulders that feels like the neck is the epicenter here. The bottom line is pain may travel, and this can make it tricky to find the true cause.

We've talked about the anatomy of the neck and how each part can become a pain in the neck. Let's go over the things we can do to prevent this and how to get back to feeling good.

Any belly sleepers out there? Sleeping on your stomach is comfy, especially in the winter, when it keeps your organs warm as they press against the bed. The drawback is that to sleep on your stomach, you have to crane your neck to the side. This can cause a bone to go out of place. (People call it a "kink" in your neck.)

And what about the supertaskers that drive, talk on the phone, fix their makeup, and have a snack all at the same time? Not only are they a danger to the road, they're probably cradling the phone between their shoulder and ear. That can really strain the muscles in your neck. What makes it worse is we usually use the same ear every time we are on the phone. This imbalance is a recipe for trouble.

Another way we mistreat our neck is if we look up or down all day long, straining our muscles by not giving them a rest every now and then. The solution is to stretch and strengthen your body. Everybody can get hurt or get sick, but if you are strong and limber, you're less likely to get injured and more likely to get better quickly. This is the armor you protect yourself with and the internal health insurance you can take to cover yourself. Whether you go all out and start up your own yoga practice or just get going with some simple stretches at your desk, it's important to just get started.

When treating the aches and pains, the question of should I use ice or heat often comes up. Ice is a good way to calm down all that inflammation in your neck. Heat can relax sore muscles, but heat can be a little tricky. If you have an area that's inflamed and you apply heat to it, you're bringing more blood to the area, which just makes the condition worse. When you go out in the sun, your face turns red because the heat causes more blood to run to your hot face. If you apply a hot pad to an inflamed neck, that heat might feel good while it's on your neck—heat can have a pleasant, numbing effect—but in the long run, your healing time will increase. So when in doubt, I recommend ice for twenty minutes at a time with forty minute breaks in between.

If you have a pain in the neck and it's not going away, there are people out there who can help. If a muscle is at the heart of the problem, a massage may be in order here. (I really had to twist your arm for that suggestion, right?) A physical therapist can get you started on a stretching and strengthening program, and a chiropractor can restore motion and get your neck lined up like it's supposed to be. People often feel betrayed by their bodies when things aren't running like a well-oiled machine. With all the abuse, wear, and tear we put our bodies through, we should really be marveling at how often our body gets it right.

Plantar Fasciitis: Walking on Pins and Needles

Folks with plantar fasciitis have a hard time getting out of bed in the morning. Not because they are lazy or tired. It's not from "one too many" the night before, or from too few zzz during sleep. It's because those with *plantar fasciitis* know that when their feet hit the ground, intense heel pain will soon follow. After a long night's rest, the first few steps of the day can be the worst.

Let's define our terminology first. The "plantar" surface is the bottom of the foot. "Fascia" is a type of tissue that holds things together. In this case it's supporting the bones in the arch of your feet. I like to think of fascia as thick plastic wrap like the kind used to save leftovers. The "itis" part lets us know the tissue is inflamed. When this tissue gets inflamed, it contracts overnight, while the foot is resting. The first steps of the day stretch out the irritated tissue, and this is what causes the burning or stabbing pain that is usually felt on the inside bottom of the foot just in front of your heel. Once the fascia is limber, the pain goes away, only to come back after the next break.

So you may be wondering who gets this condition. The weekend warriors make up the first group, those who give their feet physical overload in little spurts. Heavy activity without much muscle to support it can sometimes be too much for the feet to handle.

The next group includes people without much of an arch in their feet. They are considered flat-footed and are more prone to plantar fasciitis because arches act as shock absorbers; without them, your entire foot (not to mention knees) must hit the ground. If you consider how many steps we take in a day, this can add up to quite a beating. Imagine jumping in the water with your body straight versus a loud, slapping belly flop. With no arches in your feet, your entire foot has to smack the ground all at once. Just as a belly flop leaves you with a sore tummy, no arch support can make for a very unhappy foot.

Finally, those with arthritis and diabetes are especially prone, and bad shoes can cause it, too.

The cure really depends on what caused it. If you just bought a new pair of heels, the pain should subside once you go back to your old, supportive tennis shoes. You may have to discontinue heavy physical activity for a while. Stretching your calf muscles will take the pressure off the foot, and besides, you should be stretching every day as a matter of course.

Sometimes your heel bone gets knocked out of place; if that's what the trouble is, you can have your chiropractor put it back in. A physical therapist can instruct you on specific exercises to help strengthen the foot, and as with any inflammation, ice is always key. Three to four times a day for twenty minutes at a time will help calm them down. As we've said before, you may think that soaking your tootsies in a nice hot tub would do some good, but in fact it just aggravates the situation.

Poison Oak

Ever hear the one about the unhappy camper who happened to pick the wrong leaf to wipe with when using the great outdoor latrine? Poison oak grows like a weed because it is one, and most of us are hypersensitive to its oil when it lands on our skin.

Poison ivy, poison oak, and sumac all contain the same secret ingredient: an oil called *urushiol*. Urushiol comes from a Japanese word meaning lacquer, which seems appropriate for the oil inside this plant. To get the oil on your skin, the leaves of the plant have to be crushed or cut in some way. Tromping through the forest can be enough. And the bad news is that urushiol has a shelf life that could compete with Twinkies. In a dry environment, this oil can remain allergenic for years. This means that if some oil got on your tent from last year's camping trip, your unfriendly guest will be going camping with you again. This is why it's so important to wash your gear.

How much of this oil is needed for a reaction? About a billionth of a gram is all it takes. Translation: just a tiny bit more than nothing. A lucky 10 percent of the population is not allergic to urushiol … for now. While they may be trouble free today, this can change. Even if you've been exposed to poison oak 100 times with no ill effects, it might be your 101st that becomes the straw that breaks the camel's back. Another quirk is that your body can be more or less sensitive from season to season.

The rash usually shows up within a day or two after exposure. It may look like it's spreading, but after you've washed, it won't spread on you or anyone else. The reason for the spreading rash is that your skin absorbs the oil at different rates. To keep urushiol at bay, wash up as quickly as you can. *Tecnu soap* can really be a lifesaver here. It takes about an hour to baste into your skin, so try to beat the clock. Use cool water to shower; warm water opens your pores and invites the poison in. Also, keep an eye on your faithful sidekick, Fido. After your dog has taken a stroll and picks up some oil on his fur, it won't affect him, but it can get on you and your furniture.

If you think you've had an encounter of the three-leaf kind, here's what to do. After the blisters have begun to bubble up and you have soaped up all you can, it's time for damage control. You don't need Mom around to remind you that calamine lotion can soothe. Cool baths and compresses are also great. And speaking of tubs, soak in some oats. Oatmeal can do wonders. Baking soda paste can also relieve the itch. Long after the rash is gone, the memory of it will stay a sore spot. Hopefully this memory will serve you well, and you'll keep this oil at arm's length. And remember the trusty saying, "Leaves of three: let them be."

Prostate Enlargement

"How's your prostate, Harry?"

"It's pretty good; and yours?"

"Mine's a little robust, but I'm working on it."

The prostate and problems with its size is not a conversation men engage in often. I'm not sure why this is, but it's probably a lot like discussing trouble they might have peeing or, worse yet, difficulties with sex.

Prostate enlargement is incredibly common, and the good news is that you can help shrink it down to size. The prostate gland sits like a bead on a necklace surrounding the urethra. The urethra is the pipe a man's urine passes through. You may remember from Reproduction 101 that fluid from the prostate bathes the sperm and makes a new life possible. During its lifetime, a prostate normally grows from the size of a pea to the size of a walnut. This expansion can sometimes give the urethra a squeeze like a boa constrictor, and you can start to feel the pinch.

So how common is prostate enlargement? If a few guys go out to lunch and they can order off the senior menu, chances are good that someone will have prostate enlargement. About half of men in their sixties have this growing problem, and the numbers just skyrocket after that. Prostate enlargement is up to 90 percent for men in their seventies and eighties. Men with benign prostate enlargement have to go often, and when they do, it's difficult to get the stream going. They have difficulty emptying the bladder, which can lead to urinary tract infections. In more advanced cases, one might notice blood in their urine. If you have these symptoms, it good to go to a health-care professional to rule out more serious options.

Now, what can you do? Limiting alcohol and caffeine is a good start. Inactivity causes the body to retain urine, so keep it moving and be active. You also want to steer clear of over-the-counter decongestants, which cause the urethra to tighten as one of their side effects. The *saw palmetto* herb has been helping men with enlarged prostates for ages. Saw palmetto is extracted from the ripened berries of the saw palmetto shrub. How it does its magic is that it stops testosterone from breaking down into a hormone that causes the prostate to grow. There are always medical options, including medicine, surgery, and heat therapy.

You can always ignore the problem. But if the problem is your health, you're really just ignoring yourself. Now *that's* embarrassing!

Sweating Buckets

Remember back in junior high school gym class, doing square dancing of all things? Can this really be a sport? Isn't there already enough humiliation for a thirteen-year-old? You "do-si-do" across the stinky hall and nervously grab the hand of someone of the opposite sex and realize that it's not just the gym floor that's shiny slick.

Sweaty hands (or sweaty anything else for that matter) can be embarrassing, but our built-in air conditioners do serve a purpose. Sweat comes from hardworking muscles or nerves in overdrive. If we get hot, nervous, or get in some time at the gym, on come the water works. If you live in a relatively cool area, your body can produce about one liter per hour. If you live in a hot climate, you can sweat two to three liters an hour. For those new to the desert, it would take your body about six weeks to catch up.

Ever wonder why you are so much hotter in an area that's humid as opposed to a dry climate? It's the sweat evaporating from your skin that causes you to chill out. When it's humid outside, the water vapor in the air is near saturation. So the sweat stays trapped, dripping down your face, and you're stuck burning up.

The sweat from your underarms is different from the sweat the rest of your skin makes. Over most of your body it's just salty water mixed with a few impurities, which oozes out of your pores. The sweat from your armpits has fatty acids and proteins in it, presenting a delicious treat for the bacteria living on your skin. It may be hard to believe, but armpit sweat itself is odorless. The smell comes from the bacteria feasting on this fatty sweat. So deodorants don't work because they stop you from sweating. They work because they are acidic—meaning that the acid kills off the bacteria.

Your body can short circuit and make too much or too little sweat. Hormones (ask a woman who is going through menopause), medications, and an overactive thyroid can make you feel like you're living in a sauna. The body will hold back on sweating if you're dehydrated or during a heatstroke.

The smell of the sweat can also be a clue. Sweat that smells fruity is sometimes a sign of diabetes. An ammonia smell can signal kidney or liver disease. Sweating when you're not hot or nervous is usually sign of illness. For those Sweaty Betty's out there, everything from Botox to surgery to remove the sweat gland in your pits is up for the taking. Using a natural deodorant and bathing and wearing natural fabrics that allow your skin to breathe can do wonders. And just know that when you do sweat, it's your body working hard to keep you cool.

My What Sharp Teeth You Have

It's the middle of the night. The silence is broken by an eerie, high-pitched sound. It's the sound of bone grinding on bone. No, you're not stuck in some Hitchcock movie; it's your sleep partner grinding teeth, also known as *bruxism*. Bruxism can bring more trouble than waking up people. Sometimes it can show up in a stressful situation during the day, but it is most common at night.

How can you tell you grind your teeth if your sleep partner does not tell you? Look in the mirror. Teeth that have been worked on for a long time are worn down, sharp and flattened, or chipped. You may also be able to see the inside of your tooth from the worn-down tooth enamel. You may find yourself waking up with a dull headache, an earache, or a pain in your jaw. When things get really bad, you can wake up with a chewed-up inner cheek.

So why do some people grind when others do not? It could be that their upper and lower teeth aren't lined up right because the jaw is out of place, but more often than not, as with many health issues, stress is usually a player. People who grind during the day are better able to pinpoint the things that are causing their frustration.

We all hold our tension in different places. For some it's the gut, and they can get a stomachache when the tension hits. For grinders, it can be a physical way to express anger. Teeth grinding can also be a side effect from antidepressant medications.

How big a problem this is depends on how much a person grinds. Kids can go through a stage of teeth grinding that only lasts for a short while. It is important to mention this to your dentist. He can look out for damage to your teeth and also get you fitted for a mouth guard.

This won't help you win any popularity contests but will protect your teeth. A chiropractor can put the jawbone back in place if it is offtrack a bit, and a good massage therapist will release the tight soft tissue in and around your mouth.

All this releasing of stress in the body is pretty fruitless if you just let it build back up without addressing it. For some, this means seeing a professional; for others, they may just need a good outlet to relieve the stress … such as exercise, meditation, or a good friend to talk to.

Chapter Two:
Conditions & Syndromes

In order to change we must be sick and tired of being sick and tired.

~Author Unknown

Stress: What a GAS

Some people say that we're evolving on an exponential curve, that we will see more changes in our lifetime than in every other previous lifetime put together. What this means is that the information just keeps on coming, and this causes stress.

We know what stress is and how it feels, but do we know how it affects us? Having a nervous meltdown before a test is a normal reaction; that surge of adrenaline while walking down a dark alley at night keeps us alert. Both are natural, healthy responses to our world. On the other hand, if our stress reactions are extreme, unusual, or long-lasting, our health will begin to deteriorate.

Stress can affect each person differently and in many differing ways. Biochemical, neurological, physiological, and psychological changes occur in the body during stress. Each person has a personal stress threshold, meaning that there is no standard by which stress can be measured. What one person thrives on may be way too much stimulation for another.

People can exceed their comfort levels and experience *dis*-stress when excessive, prolonged, and/or extreme stress puts the body into General

Adaptation Syndrome (GAS). This syndrome is the beginning of a long and slippery slope of symptoms, which may include fatigue, high or low blood sugar, high cholesterol, anxiety, depression, insomnia, headaches, and bad breath. One reason that the symptoms are so varied is that distress affects the weakest link in a person's biochemical makeup, amplifying preexisting problems or conditions. The first organ that stress affects are the adrenal glands, which is very sensitive to stress in all forms, including stimulants such as coffee, alcohol, and tobacco.

There are three stages of stress: (1) alarm-fight or flight, (2) maintenance, and (3) exhaustion. The alarm stage brings on the rapid adrenal response, flooding the body with adrenalin and creating the "rush" one gets when startled or frightened. Our adrenal glands were designed to work in this manner to protect us from danger.

The maintenance stage is a by-product of life-in-fast-lane living, where the adrenal glands are constantly depleted from perpetual on-the-go (flight or fight) responses to stressful stimuli. Symptoms at this stage include difficulty sleeping, chronic fatigue, and susceptibility to subtle toxemias such as allergies; low resistance to illness, leading to frequent colds and infections; and emotional instability due to hormonal changes. Pain and inflammatory complexes (arthritis variations) may develop as the body loses the ability to make proper levels of cortisone and other anti-inflammatory hormones. More and more people are in this phase of GAS due to the rapid rate of information/stimulation talked about at the beginning of the article.

In exhaustion, the final stage of GAS, the body actually begins to shut down in order to slow the person. Along with the ever-present fatigue, the person may also experience depression and anxiety; disease processes may begin to manifest.

Because stress and its ramifications are so prevalent today, we check the adrenals as part of a regular chiropractic visit using a simple muscle test. Along with clearing the nervous system with adjustments, we often recommend nutritional supplements to support the adrenals as well as whatever other systems are weakened. Simple lifestyle modifications can help prevent stress:

- eat whole foods
- avoid foods high in sodium
- select foods high in potassium
- avoid refined foods, sugar, alcohol, and caffeine
- get sufficient sleep
- practice some sort of relaxation
- drink plenty of filtered water every day
- recognize stressors and don't ignore them
- enjoy natural sunlight
- get adjusted regularly

Can't Sit Still

After the fifth trip to the principal's office, Billy was sent home with a note recommending that he needed to get checked for ADD. *ADD*, or *attention deficit disorder* is a syndrome that is characterized by short attention span, impulsiveness, and often hyperactivity. It's the kid who can't sit still, who talks out of turn, whose grades reflect poor concentration skills.

Teachers are often the first to suggest this possible diagnosis, but the path from suggestion to the child being given drugs for ADD is often way too short. Eager parents often enter the doctor's office with their minds made up and look at the appointment as the place to get their prescription written when other considerations for a child's misbehavior should be looked at first.

The jury is still out on the safety of stimulant drugs prescribed for ADD. The problem is that it's the drug companies that finance most of the research on the syndrome. These companies benefit from positive results. Those against drug treatment for ADD point to animal research. These studies show that the frontal lobe of the animal's brain becomes sluggish and its enthusiasm for life diminishes. Let's hope that's not true for humans.

What everyone would agree is that it is important to avoid misdiagnosing an unruly kid as ADD and giving prescription drugs the child doesn't need. How many of us acted out in class? Imagine someone labeling you as a small child with ADD, telling you that you have a problem and need to take drugs to be normal. That's why it's so important to be careful.

So what do you do if your kid's teacher says he or she may have ADD? A good first step is a general health exam for anemia, hearing and visual acuity deficiencies, hypothyroidism and other possible health problems, any of which may be the underlying cause. After those alternatives have been checked out, an applied kinesiologist can look for *neurological disorganization*. This can be explained quite simply. Say you missed the crawling stage as an infant. Crawling helps the nervous system develop bilaterally. You go on to the next stage without being ready. It's like being in an algebra class not knowing basic math.

If your child only has ADD in certain situations, like at school, it's probably not ADD. A child with ADD has ADD all the time. Consider the situation. If he acts up at school, particularly after lunch, what he's eating could be the problem. If french fries are the only vegetable available in the lunchroom, the child's blood-sugar level might be all over the board. Only a physician can diagnose ADD, and it's important to have it addressed. Just make sure you've taken the time your kid deserves to be sure the assumed diagnosis is right.

There Is no Such Thing as Cellulite

I bet that got your attention even if you have personal evidence to argue against this statement. The word "cellulite" was actually made up by those who make money claiming to rid the body of this obtrusive invader. To the body, fat is fat and that's that. Fat can be stored in your muscles like marbled meat, but your body places most of your fat just under your skin. This means that when your legs look like orange peel, it does not mean that something strange is brewing under the surface of your skin.

For most of us, our knowledge of cellulite or why we have fat on our bodies is pretty limited. So let's make a temporary truce with our enemy and learn more about fat. We all have fat and we all need fat. Anytime we eat more calories than we are using, the body will save it for a rainy day. Dining on a fat-free diet won't save you either. Unless you're eating that 300-calorie fat-free bar while running on the treadmill, your body will find a place to store it. And food manufacturers can usually be counted on put extra salt or something else you don't need into their fat-free creations to make up for the flavor lost from removing the fat.

Once puberty is over, the final tally on the number of fat cells you have in your body is fixed. People with more fat cells tend to gain weight faster. While the number of solders in your fat army stays the same, the growth in size of each one is unlimited. Once these fat cells reach a certain girth, that infamous rippling over the skin can happen. So you can never really lose fat cells; the best you can do is shrink their size.

If our body is so smart, why can't it not just get rid of what we don't use? Our bodies were made to survive the harsh times when food is hard to come by. In today's world of super Wal-marts and cheese that's "good" for a year, that time never comes. The extra something we carry ends up as a permanent extra all year round.

We know there are many problems from being too fat, but what about being too thin? For women, infertility is a possibility. We need fat to make estrogen, and when levels fall, so will our chances of getting pregnant. Fat also protects our internal organs like the heart and brain. It is also the body's insulation keeping us warm at night. Without fat, vitamins A, D, E, and K would not have a place to hide out in the body.

The more we learn about the human body, the more we find to respect. And even if we don't like it, the body is smart to store fat. We just have to use the same good sense when we choose what we nourish it with.

The Dreaded Earache

Ear infections, or *otitis media*, are the most common cause of pediatric visits and subsequent antibiotic use during the first two years of a child's life. In fact, they account for over 50 percent of all visits to pediatricians.

An earache is an infection that causes an inflammation or swelling of the middle ear. Younger children are more susceptible to earaches because their eustachian tubes are smaller in diameter and more horizontal than in later years, but anyone of any age can get an ear infections.

A child with an acute earache will most probably have had a cold, sore throat, sinusitis, or some other type of upper respiratory infection. They may be reacting to an allergy as well. Symptoms include a possible fever and the trademark red, bulging eardrum.

Traditional treatment for ear infections is to prescribe antibiotics, despite the lack of evidence of their effectiveness. In some studies, children who were given antibiotics actually experienced increased recurrences compared to children who were given placebo treatments. This may be a result of the suppressive effects that antibiotics have on the immune systems and their disturbance of the normal flora of the upper respiratory tract.

When medication does not work, surgery is performed, inserting a tiny plastic tube to assist drainage. One million American children have this surgery each year, despite reports by the *Journal of the American Medical Association* that assert that just 42 percent of these surgeries are appropriate.

The causes for earache are not always known, but many risk factors have been well documented: day-care attendance promotes the spread of just about everything, including the pathogens involved with ear infections; early exposure to secondhand smoke or the smoke from wood-burning stoves can lead to abnormal ear tube function; food allergies have been identified as causal in as many as 93 percent of children with chronic earaches.

Prevention is the best cure for an earache. Breastfed babies have been shown to be less likely to get ear infections than bottle-fed babies. This may be due to the protective qualities in human milk that guard against infection in general and/or potential allergens in cow's milk. Breast-feeding for a minimum of the first four months enhances the baby's immune system. Babies who have been breastfed have thymus glands twenty times larger than those of their formula-fed counterparts; the thymus gland is the major organ involved in the immune system in children.

Avoiding foods that small children are commonly allergic to can also prevent earaches. It is advisable to avoid fowl, dairy, wheat, eggs, and peanuts during the first nine months of life. Taking the precaution of feeding the baby different foods rather than consistently feeding the same type of any food is also a good way to prevent allergy development. Rotating minimizes the likelihood that the child will become oversensitive to one food or food group.

Taking thymus gland extract, though not vegan friendly, can help improve immune function and is great in treating earaches. Humidifiers have been a popular preventive measure as well; though scientists are still unsure why they work, the fact remains that they do. Ninety-three percent of all patients who receive chiropractic care alone see improvement within the first week of treatments that release the physical stress on the central nervous system.

When your little one gets an earache, remember to get it properly diagnosed, and let your decision for treatment be an educated one. You should visit your physician, just as you would for any potentially serious threat.

The Pain of Fibromyalgia

Have you ever had that pesky check engine light go off in your car? You dutifully take it to mechanic after mechanic, only to be told there's nothing wrong. Even after all the tests tell you everything's fine, that light just won't go off.

Fibromyalgia is a lot like that light. All the X-rays, MRIs, and blood work tell you everything's dandy, but your body tells a totally different story. So let's try to set the story straight.

What does fibromyalgia feel like? Think back to the last time you had the flu. Remember that achy feeling all over your body? Your muscles felt overworked and stiff, and your body was in a constant yearning for siesta. You felt tired but had trouble getting a good night's sleep … like your body had come unplugged from its power supply. These are the basic symptoms. Some sufferers add headaches, sensitivity to light and odors, and abdominal pain to the list. To make matters worse, in order to be labeled for diagnosis, your symptoms must be felt for at least three months in at least eleven different spots in the body.

Finding out what causes fibromyalgia has been a tricky. Some have guessed that stress is involved, because stressful situations seem to ignite flair-ups. Others think hormones might be involved, because the condition is mainly found in women. At the head of the pack is a theory called *central sensitization*. Like a short circuit, the brain's perception of pain goes haywire. The body overreacts in response to pain signals, so a tap on the shoulder might be perceived as a real hammering for someone with fibromyalgia. Since all pain is felt in the brain, this pain feels as real as any other.

Treatment for fibromyalgia can be just as tricky as the diagnosis and cause. It's one of those conditions where the word "management" is used instead of "cure," meaning that you're in it for the long haul. Some turn to medicine to manage the symptoms. Their doctors might prescribe muscle relaxants or antidepressants. Many look outside of the box, turning to chiropractic care or acupuncture to try to get back to balance. Others have also found relief on the massage table.

A key to healing here is having the support of those around you. This disease is often dismissed because it can't be seen on an X-ray or under a microscope. For someone to help you with this, they first need to understand that the pain is real. Those with fibromyalgia can help themselves by keeping their lives as stress-free as possible and eating healthy, organic, whole foods.

Your body gets to decide how it gets sick. You can decide how to help it get well.

Hemochromatosis: Iron Overload

You're out grocery shopping, looking for a good cereal. One boasts that it's fortified with iron, and you drop it into the cart. You can never get enough iron, right? It's a key ingredient in blood, and your immune system is shot without it.

This is true for most people, but for those with hereditary *hemochromatosis,* iron overload can literally poison the body. Hemochromatosis is a disease whose signs do not show up until midlife. The challenge is that early symptoms—which may include arthritis, fatigue, abdominal pain, and lack of sex drive—can easily be misdiagnosed as a symptom of some other problem or condition.

For people with hemochromatosis, their bodies absorb higher percentages of iron than normal—normal being roughly 10 percent while those with hemochromatosis take in as much as 20 percent—and stash it away for a rainy day, stockpiling more iron than the body would ever need. Over the years, these quantities can lead to toxic overload.

Although the extra iron gets stored in all the major organs, the liver is the favorite hot spot. In advanced hemochromatosis, the liver will suffer the most damage, in some cases leading to cirrhosis, liver failure, or cancer of the liver. A hallmark of this stage is that the person's skin will turn a bronze color due to all the excess iron.

So now that I've got your attention with all the scary possibilities, you may be wondering how you get this disease. It is an inherited genetic mutation, which means that you're born with its potential written in your blueprints. Screening is available to see if you have the gene, however not everyone with the mutation develops symptoms. So you could test positive for something that may never affect you.

People usually find out that they have it through a simple blood/iron test after some of the symptoms have popped up and after many other conditions have been ruled out.

The good news is that it's easy to test for; the better news is that it's really easy to treat. The ancient practice of bloodletting actually did some good in cases like this, and doctors continue to prescribe it today. Nowadays, it's called phlebotomy, and it involves donating about a pint of blood a week to save the sufferer from serious complications. Your doctor will ask you to stop taking iron supplements or foods high in iron. Vitamin C is also to be avoided because it aids in the absorption of iron. Our bodies are working hard all the time to defend you from toxins and menacing bugs. So I consider the body the best doctor of all. Listen to what it has to tell you. The messages it sends are worthy of your undivided attention.

Irritable Bowel Syndrome

Whether we care to admit it or not, we've all had diarrhea and we've all been constipated. On the runny end of things, it's our body's way of getting rid of something we should have steered clear of in the first place. When things get stuck, this is a clear signal that the body needs a little more fiber to get the traffic to pick up the pace and move along.

For the one in five Americans whose bodies are switching gears all the time, they spend little or no time going with the regular flow. *Irritable bowel syndrome* (IBS) is what happens when a person has bouts of diarrhea and constipation that last at least twelve weeks.

Yikes! Twelve weeks???

Surprising to many, but it's true. And yet IBS is so common that it should be as familiar to us as a fever or the flu. Why don't we know much about it? For the simple reason that no one wants to talk about the issues they have with their intestines or hear about them from someone else.

Your body has a natural rhythm. Muscles in the body that maintain the machine's vital organs, like the ones in your heart and lungs, work nonstop, even when you're asleep. They don't need our attention to do their jobs.

There are equally important muscles that line our intestines. Working like a well-oiled assembly line, these muscles contract and relax, moving food down your pipes as your body takes what it needs and discards the rest. If this system moves too fast, as in the case of diarrhea, your body does not have time to remove all the vital nutrients. If we slow it down, as in the case of constipation, the body takes out a toxin or two. In either case, the result can be very painful, leaving the person feeling bloated and adding abdominal cramping, gas, and the social and emotional awkwardness that accompany them. To make matters worse, diarrhea and constipation can irritate hemorrhoids.

IBS is a syndrome, which means that the exact cause is not medically known. It also means that there are no specific tests that identify it. So problems like lactose intolerance and celiac disease need to be ruled out, which means that diagnosis is largely done using the process of elimination (no pun intended).

So what are the treatment options with IBS? Some people approach the problem with fiber or antidiarrheal medication to try to balance the pendulum, but if they're not careful, they can end up swinging it too far the other way. The excess fiber makes them constipated and vice versa.

Sometimes it is a malfunctioning *ileocecal* valve, and a good chiropractor can check that. In many cases, it is likely that your diet plays a role. A nutritionalist may ask a patient to keep a food journal to uncover what "triggers" the episodes. Stress can also effect digestion, so finding an outlet to let go of that toxic energy is essential. Try yoga, massage, meditation, or whatever works for you.

Diet is what you put in your mouth and that's your choice. But it's nutrition that really matters, and nutrition is what your body decides to take from the options given.

Is Your Mouth Bone-Dry?

Looking at a baby who is teething, you may think all that saliva running down their chin is kind of gross. The bib area of their clothes is always wet, and everything is getting slobbered on. It's hard to imagine years down the road when there might be a lack of saliva, as many adults have.

Xerostomia, or dry mouth, is very common, especially in our aging adult communities. It is all too often ignored and all too easy to repair to justify this lack of attention.

The big deal is that with xerostomia, you have a better chance of getting cavities, because saliva helps remove all that build-up that occurs between brushings. It is essential for healthy teeth and gums, and what's more, minerals found in saliva can actually repair early tooth decay.

You can get little sores at the corners of your mouth, which can be painful especially when you open your mouth wide. And your breath may cause others to take a step back. A lack of saliva can make it difficult to talk. It even can change the way things taste. And don't forget that saliva is a part of the digestive system, which means that without it, we're sending food down the tube that's not ready for departure.

We are supposed to produce about three liters of saliva a day. When production slows down, it's sometimes a factor of age. The sensors for thirst in our brain can wear down; the glands that make the saliva can also get lethargic. But more often than not, it's the contents of your medicine cabinet that are to blame. Antihistamines, high blood pressure medication, depression medication, muscle relaxants, and thousands of other pills can make your mouth dry up.

Dry mouth itself may also be a symptom of a disease. Your body may be telling you of a problem with your endocrine system or depression, among other possibilities.

What to do about this depends on what causes it. If medication is to blame, make sure you tell the doctor who prescribed it. The doctor may change your prescription or your dosage. Until you sort it all out, it's even more important to keep your pearly whites clean, so brush often and drink lots of water. A good trick to increase the amount of water you drink is to keep a bottle or glass with you. You'll find yourself sipping at it the entire day, and your body will benefit. A humidifier by your bed will help keep your mouth moist through the night.

And if you don't know why your mouth is dry, you should go to a qualified heath provider to get to the bottom of it. Our body is constantly giving us clues to our general health. We can choose to ignore them, but then we cannot say we were not warned.

Nosebleeds

Ever wonder about nosebleeds? What is the best way to turn that bloody hydrant off? And why does it bleed like that in the first place? Sure we can blame the pickers, but there are plenty of ear scratchers and eye rubbers out there, and we never see them running for the bathroom to grab a tissue to soak up the flood. The nose has many tiny blood vessels lying close to the outside surface of our skin that work hard to warm and add moisture to the air that we breathe. Their close proximity to the surface also makes them more prone to injury.

Why are some bleeders and others not? The biggest culprit is the gold digger equipped with sharp, intruding tools. Dry air also does it, causing the vessels to work overtime. Colds, allergies, and a sucker punch can also do the trick. More serious causes include clotting problems due to aspirin therapy and hypertension.

Okay, we know how it starts, how do we get it to stop? The first instruction is: don't panic. Surges of adrenalin will only increase the hemorrhaging. Next, it's a good idea to lean slightly forward while sitting up. Sitting up keeps gravity on your side, and leaning forward keeps you from swallowing your own blood. Blood sliding down your throat can cause nausea, vomiting, and diarrhea. (As if you didn't have enough to deal with!)

To stop the flow, there are now two main strategies: You can pinch your nose for about ten minutes or until all is clear; or you can cut out the source by applying pressure to the major blood vessel to the nose. Find some wet cotton (or tissue) and place it where your upper lip meets your gums, then use your fingers to apply some upward pressure against the cotton. When done correctly this trick works faster than the nose pinching.

For chronic bleeders, there are some additional steps you can take. For little ones, keep their fingernails short. They might fess up to the picking if you ask, "Which finger do you pick with?" rather than, "Do you pick?" If dry air is the guilty party, a humidifier in the dry months will do the trick. Open your mouth when you sneeze, no matter what Molly Manners might say. Cover your mouth, of course, but don't sneeze though your nose.

And, if you needed to hear another reason to avoid tobacco, cigarettes can dry out the nose and cause nosebleeds. If you get them often and can't figure out why, you might want to tell your health-care provider. It could be anything from a pill you're taking to your blood being under too much pressure. Taking care of you in little everyday ways will add up to a higher quality life.

Thoracic Outlet Syndrome

Our blood vessels and nerves map out a freeway around our body. In the blink of an eye, blood circulates to every cell before heading back to the heart, and your brain sends signals along your nervous system highway from its perch at central command. There are snags and traffic jams every once in a while. Just like rush hour on a big city freeway, there are parts of the body where blood vessels and nerves get squeezed into a congested area, and the next thing you know there's a real snarl up.

One of these areas in the body is the space between the collarbone and your first rib. When traffic is bumper-to-bumper, it becomes something named thoracic outlet syndrome.

The space between your collarbone and the first rib, which sits just behind it, is a snug place that normally manages to accommodate the nerves and blood vessels that travel this pathway to and from the arm. When thoracic outlet syndrome occurs, this space becomes compromised.

We find this happening for many reasons. It can happen as a result of an accident, for example. In car accidents, the seatbelt often pushes the collarbone back with considerable force. Years of dropping your shoulders (bad posture) can put on the squeeze. Those big purses that hold everything but the kitchen sink can contribute to the problem; so can those backpacks that are as big as (or bigger) than the kid carrying it.

We can also be set up for it through our genetic makeup. Normally, we only have ribs branching off our thoracic vertebrae, but some of us are born with a small rib coming off our lowest bone in our neck. This extra bone can sit right in the middle of the action. Any or all of these things can compromise the nerves and vessels in the area.

And what does thoracic outlet syndrome feels like? It really depends on what is being pinched. If the nerves (the *brachial plexus*) are feeling the squeeze, the messages between your brain and your arm are going to go haywire, manifesting as numbness or an electric shock–like pain in the shoulder, arm, or hand. You might experience difficulty opening jars from a weakened grip.

If a blood vessel is being pinched, you might notice some swelling in your hand and possibly the hand hungry for blood might begin to look a little blue.

With thoracic outlet syndrome, you could wait around and hope it goes away. But life is short, and there's also a possibility of permanent damage out there. Chiropractors can often get to the bottom of things and take the pressure off the nerves and vessels.

You might also want to look at your posture and keep your shoulders back. A good massage might be in order, too. When your body turns on the "check engine" light, it's time to pop the hood and do a little body maintenance.

Scoliosis

Of the many places that you may want an extra curve in your body, your back is not one of them. When looking at a person straight on, his or her backbone should line up perfectly straight, with each bone stacked and centered above the one below. The lumbar curve, or the natural curve in your neck, should be visible in profile only. In other words, your spine should curve front to back, not from side to side.

Scoliosis can be easy to spot if you know where to look. It usually begins in early adolescence, which is also the time that kids become self-conscious and tend to cover up more, making early detection difficult. It almost always begins painlessly, so don't count on your kids to complain of back pain to find out if something is wrong.

The pelvis, shoulders, and head should all be level—this can be easily checked by looking in a mirror. The shoulder blades can be a great place to look, too. They should be equal distance from the spine and should not flare or "wing" out. A typical red flag will be one shoulder blade that does not look like the other. In addition, with scoliosis, muscles in the low back can get a ropey appearance on one side. When the child bends over and touches her toes, one side of the back should not be higher than the other. If you suspect that your child may have scoliosis, have it checked out by a qualified professional.

Why is early detection so important? If the problem is not corrected or the progression at least slowed in the early stages, irreversible changes take place. Backbones are normally block-shaped, and after years of unequal pressure from scoliosis, the bones can become wedge-shaped, like a slice of pizza. The ribs that are connected to these wedge-shaped bones also adapt to this curve, making it impossible to correct.

Teenagers grow fast and so can the angle of the curve in their backs. Scoliosis can lead to a lot more than bad posture. Unchecked, it can lead to severe back pain, difficulty breathing, deformity, and in extreme cases, injury to the heart and lungs.

Most cases of scoliosis are caused by an imbalance of the muscular support to the spine due to poor nerve control. The muscles attached to the spine become tighter on one side of the back than the other.

A medical doctor would monitor for changes, use a brace if the curve got bad, and recommend surgery if the curve was greater than 40 to 50 degrees. While surgery is not usually necessary, a curve this acute can have serious consequences if left untreated.

Chiropractors work on restoring the natural neurological and muscular balance to allow the backbone to straighten itself the best it can. Massage may also be necessary to restore balance. The worst treatment for possible scoliosis in an adolescent would be to ignore it, so if you suspect that it might be an issue, have it checked by your health-care provider.

Chapter Three:
Behaviors

*Diseases of the soul are more dangerous and more
numerous than those of the body.*

~ Cicero

Detox: Not Just for Addicts

People have been fasting since the dawn of history. I'm not talking
about starving during hard times but purposely reducing your caloric
intake for a specific reason. The most common use of fasting, I'd guess,
is for detoxification or to cleanse the body. By reducing the amount
and types of food we take in, we allow our body's systems to rest and,
often, to release stored toxins. When the body isn't so busy dealing with
all the stuff coming it, it will take the opportunity and clean house.

We are increasingly exposed to more and more toxins in our everyday
life. Along with the usual suspects like environmental toxins, including
pollution, pesticides, and secondhand smoke, we are also subjected to
internal toxins. These include bacteria and parasites, candida, drugs,
and metabolic wastes. Some of the toxic danger we're exposed to is
not so obvious. For instance, even though DDT was banned in this
country, we still export it and then import the food grown in the
contaminated soil.

The National Academy of Sciences estimates the average American
ingestion of pesticides such as DDT (in food sources alone) to be around
40 mg per year, and also estimates that we carry about 100mg stored

in body fat. You may wonder how this may affect us. It is believed that van Gogh's mental state could have resulted from lead poisoning (he licked his paintbrush). Other sources of lead include old pipes, paint, and even unfiltered water.

Bringing down the number of calories you take in can facilitate the detoxification process and allow the liver to rest, but total fasting may release the toxins from the fatty tissue too quickly. If the detox pathways are not running efficiently, released toxins are left to recirculate and redeposit in body tissues, causing pain, inflammation, and disease. For best results, cutting down the calories (without fasting) and adding a good detox supplementation to the regimen can ensure efficient removal of toxins at a pace the body can easily handle. It is also important to consult with your qualified health-care provider.

Supplements can help with your detox in many ways. Chelators bind heavy metals, antioxidants and nutrients facilitate Detox pathways, and multivitamin/mineral support provides energy and balance when caloric intake is low. A good, unsweetened protein powder can be beneficial for maintaining blood sugar, and Siberian ginseng contributes to energy and support of the adrenal glands (which also provide blood-sugar support).

It is important that the supplements address all seven detox pathways in the body: liver, bowel, blood, lungs, lymph, skin, and kidneys. All these pathways should be detoxified, and proper nutrients should be provided to ensure a slow, efficient, healthy removal of stored toxins, both environmental and internal.

Super Size Me

Obesity is growing in epidemic proportions (no pun intended). It will soon become the number-one health concern in the United States, and as our guts get larger, health-care providers are scrambling to come up with solutions.

Obesity-related diseases cost the U.S. $100 billion annually, more than the cost of smoking and problem drinking combined. Obesity is responsible for 400,000 deaths per year and significantly increases many risk factors, including heart disease, type 2 diabetes, colon and breast cancer, hypertension, gall bladder disease, and osteoarthritis. Eighty percent of obese people have one of these conditions, and nearly 40 percent have two or more.

More than 64 percent of the U.S. population is overweight. One reason is that childhood obesity has skyrocketed: the number of overweight children and teens is 15 percent. A recent study concluded that the average three-year-old spends 79 percent of the time sedentary, with less than twenty minutes in physical activity per day. In 1977, children had one fast-food meal in ten meals. By 1996, the ratio was one in three.

The debate in the health-care field is whether obesity should be classified as a disease. Classifying it as a disease would entitle doctors to be reimbursed for treating obesity with procedures like gastric bypass surgery, liposuction, or prescription drugs that lower the body mass index (BMI). Meanwhile, physicians of natural medicine are concerned that classifying obesity as a disease would remove personal control and shift the blame to someone else.

Furthermore, under this definition, exercise programs that involve the patient in proactive pursuits that lead to normal blood-glucose levels and improved cholesterol levels could be considered failures if they did not reduce weight. In truth, fitness is a much more important indicator of health outcomes than fatness, because the key in facilitating weight loss is to balance the body. Nutritional and metabolic problems can cause imbalances that make weight loss difficult, if not impossible. Sticking to healthy eating habits, exercising, correcting nutritional deficiencies, repairing metabolic dysfunction, and avoiding food allergies can foster true, long-term weight loss.

As chiropractors, we help our patients achieve optimal weight loss by helping them bring their unbalanced systems into balance. Our goal is to help patients achieve and maintain the homeostasis of many systems, including the endocrine system. Less than optimal functioning in various organs of the endocrine system will thwart efforts to bring weight into balance. The thyroid gland controls the basal metabolic rate for almost every cell in the body. The pancreas secretes insulin to bring glucose into the cell to be burned for energy. The liver uses glycogen for energy storage. The adrenal glands secrete factors that regulate blood sugar, water retention, and metabolism. Impaired function of any of these organ systems can impede weight loss.

Balancing blood sugar is essential. Sensible eating habits have less to do with willpower than they have with blood sugar. When blood sugar drops, the brain signals the body that it is in a hunger state; mental confusion and weakness generally follow. This is why starving all day to make up for the calories consumed in the evening is not a smart approach! Adding protein to a meal in the form of a supplement of protein powder can help balance blood sugar. Eliminating sugar and simple, unrefined carbohydrates will help achieve balance as well. This is the principle behind the low-carb diets. Food allergies can cause weight gain by causing edema, water weight gain, and actual weight gain by producing substances that trigger the body to store fat.

Remember, the plan that works is the plan that works for you! If your treatment plan does not take off weight and keep it off, why bother? Until you find the one you can stick to, you haven't found the right diet.

This Should Make You Sit Up Straight

What does your posture say about you? Is it whispering, "I'm tired"? Is it screaming, "I've driven 500 miles today, and I'm just trying to make it home"? How about, "I'm a teenager and not going to pay attention to you"? Our posture can say a lot about what's going on in our minds, and it offers an equally good view of what's going on with our spine as well.

Let's begin with anterior head carriage for starters. The average noggin weighs about twelve pounds. So does a bowling ball. Normally, your head should sit square just over your shoulders. Often we jut our neck forward, and our head sits in front instead of over our shoulders. Too many hours in a chat room or behind a wheel can cause this.

Here's where the importance of the bowling ball analogy comes in. It's much more difficult to hold a bowling ball out in front of you instead of right up next to your body. Your body has to do a lot more work to hold your head up when it's way out in front of you.

You can easily spot anterior head carriage on your neighbor by just catching a side view, but what about you? A quick test is to find an empty wall and back up to it. The back of your head and your shoulders should hit the wall at the same time. If your back hits first, your head is a step in front of you. If your shoulders don't hit at the same time, you could be developing a hump.

Over the long haul, the price is much higher than bruising Molly Manner's feelings. Imagine the muscles in the back of your neck working overtime to support your head as it leans forward. All this extra pressure on the discs or joints between your neck bones can translate to premature arthritis. Just picture the bones in your neck building tiny unstable bridges to brace the area.

The damage does not stop there. Poor posture slows down lymphatic drainage in the neck. And we've just looked at the neck. The entire body gets thrown for a loop when our shoulders roll forward or our beer gut rocks our pelvis forward. This means that if your body is overworking just to stand up straight, important work like healing damaged cells or keeping your hormones in balance might end up getting left behind.

How we walk is another clue to posture problems. For the average Jill or Joe, the way we carry ourselves is a clue to our mood and attitude. Through the eyes of a chiropractor, your gait reveals the way your bones stack up on the inside.

Humans are top heavy: two skinny little legs hold up our whole body. Since most of us began to use those legs around our first birthday, by the time we reach adulthood, we feel as if we've got the whole walking thing covered. But just because you've been doing it most of your life doesn't mean you've been doing it right.

A whole crew of muscles has to relax while another group contracts in order to walk, and all your muscles must take turns working in the right order. Some of us look down while we walk, straining the back of our necks. To allow our bodies to support us properly, we should be gazing about fifteen feet ahead. The *cross-crawl mechanism* is a balancing procedure that causes the opposite arm to go forward when the leg is raised. For those who don't swing our arms when we walk, our hands might swell up after a long trot. Our abdominal muscles should be active to keep our hips tucked in. For those with stiffness in the hip joint, you might not be able to swing and rotate them enough while taking a step. Those with chronically stubbed toes are suffering from a lack of clearance in their stride.

It doesn't take a mirror to reveal the truth about your posture and your gait. Your shoes can be read like a book: look at how the tread is worn down. If your shoes are balding on the insides, you might be looking at falling arches, or possibly, you're knock-kneed. Wear on the outsides of your shoes can mean a number of things, including weak ankles. If one shoe is more worn than the other, chances are that your hips are tilted. This can cause your feet to hit the ground with unequal force.

Okay, now that you're a wise walker with pretty posture, what can you do to maintain and improve? Staying conscious of your bad habits is an excellent start. Go to a chiropractor to make sure that you're all stacked up right. A yoga regimen can help achieve balance. Some therapy to repair a clipped wing might be necessary too. And crawling (of all things) for five minutes a day can help connect that left-right coordination.

You can face the day slumped over, waiting for life to happen to you, or you can stand up straight, breathe deep, and take it on your terms. It's up to you.

A Workstation that Works for You

What can cause carpel tunnel syndrome, backaches, headaches, knee injury, eyestrain, and shoulder pain among many other aches and pains? Sounds like it must be something pretty serious to cause so many problems. Well it is, and it's a workstation that does not work for you. It's the chair that's too tall, and the computer that sends a glare back at you. The world of ergonomics is huge, covering everything from lighting to the distance to the nearest bathroom, but for now we'll just cover a workstation at a desk.

First, we'll cover the chair, your throne from which you conduct your business. An ideal seat should swivel 360 degrees to avoid any twisting. Armrests, when properly adjusted, are great for relieving weight from your spine. If the seat is too deep, your lower back won't be supported by the backrest. This can cause poor posture and low back pain. (This is common for those of us shorter folks.) Your hips and knees should both form right angles. If your feet dangle in the air while sitting, you're putting pressure on your lower back. Contoured seats, while they look pretty fancy, actually limit the number of seated positions possible. Among other problems, this can lower your energy level.

Your keyboard should be right around elbow height. Bending your wrist while typing can cause carpel tunnel syndrome. A simple foam palm rest will keep the wrist in a proper natural position. Your computer should just below eye level to keep your neck happy, and a screen clipped on the monitor can get rid of some of that glare.

So, should you inform your boss you're not going to lift a finger until your new workstation arrives? I wouldn't. Look around and see what you can adjust. Try to move things around to make them work for you. If your feet don't hit the ground and your chair won't adjust, try placing a phone book under your feet. Ask your boss to work with you on the problem. Most Americans will drive themselves to work if they're not on their deathbed, so most people will be at work with a headache or wrist pain; they just won't get as much done and chances are good that they'll be pretty cranky. This means that most bosses will be more than happy to help if it means bringing peace to the workplace and improving productivity. As for picking out your own chair at home, the perfect one is one that is adjustable. One that allows you to adjust the height, armrest, and the lumbar support is best.

A workstation that is built around the person using it just makes sense. When we spend our time in unsuitable conditions, we adapt to those conditions, and the body takes the abuse.

The Seven Great Paths to ... Detox

The seven pathways that the body uses to cleanse and get rid of toxins consist of the liver, bowels, blood, lungs, lymph, skin, and kidneys. It is important to plan and prepare for a cleansing and not just wing it by going on a fast, which may bring out too many toxins too quickly.

The Liver: The liver gets first crack at our nutrients; at the same time, it also gets all the toxins we take in. Continued overload on the liver interferes with the enzymes of detoxification and can result in strain on the pancreas and digestive system. The liver uses nutrients to hook onto the toxins to make them water soluble and eliminate them.

One of the reasons that vegetables like broccoli have a reputation for being cancer preventative is that they benefit the liver's detox pathways, releasing free radicals and introducing antioxidant protection in the form of vitamins C and E, beta-carotene, and selenium.

The Bowels: Because our colon is the elimination pathway for toxins, it is important it is not obstructed. There are many nutrients that can enhance optimal function, including those high in fiber like beetroot, asparagus, and broccoli. These plants contain many phytochemicals that contribute to efficient detox and elimination.

The Blood: The blood is the main thoroughfare that connects the parts of the body. It carries cells that bind and transport waste, carries toxins to the kidneys and lungs to be eliminated, and delivers oxygen to clean and iron to feed every working part of the system. Just as the hemoglobin in human blood is considered to be the primary source of nutrition in people, chlorophyll performs a similar role in plants, transforming the sun's energy through a process called photosynthesis and turning it into fuel. Studies show that taking chlorophyll as a supplement is an excellent way to improve blood-cleaning and bacteria-scavenging activities in the blood.

The Lungs: If you've ever had a breathalyzer check to determine the presence of alcohol in your blood, you know that the lungs provide a very efficient way to dump toxins, including alcohol. The liver and the skin play a role here too. When the liver has to work overtime, we pay the price with a hangover; when the skin releases toxins, the smell of alcohol is released as well.

The Lymph: Our lymph system, including the lymph nodes, is an important part of our immune system that plays a vital role in eliminating toxins. When our body fights invasions of any sort, we may notice swollen lymph nodes. The nodes act like a way station, holding the casualties of war until they can be eliminated.

The Skin: Skin conditions that are the result of accumulated wastes can temporarily increase when backed-up wastes are released into the blood. The more aggressive the liver's detox process, the bigger the load released. The skin often shows visible (and smellable) signs of the detox process that is going on. We can sometimes see pimples or boils when a cleansing process is under way or smell alcohol on our skin after excessive drinking. When we see tangible evidence that our body is working overtime, it's a good idea to heed the wake-up call and detox slowly, using the right nutrients. "Yellow dock" is often helpful with skin conditions that arise.

The Kidney: The kidneys are like filters, pulling waste from the blood and flushing it into the urine. Drinking lots of water during cleansing helps the kidneys flush your system. Dandelion works on the kidney detox pathway as well as on the blood, liver, and colon and is valuable as a general tonic and diuretic.

All seven pathways must work together for optimal removal of toxins. This process is enhanced with vitamins, minerals, and other nutritional supplements that combine to support the body through detox and protect against cellular damage. Reducing your caloric intake, supplementing your diet with a protein power, and eating a balanced nutritional diet can optimize health and well-being by ridding the body of toxic waste. For the safest and best results, consult your chiropractor and/or health-care provider before you begin your cleanse.

Do I Use Ice or Heat?

"Hey doc, will sitting in my hot tub relieve my sciatica?"

The question of using heat or ice comes up every day in our office. Most people are ready to do their part to take care of themselves but just aren't sure where to start. Ask one person and they swear by ice. According to a hot-tub salesman, blessed relief is just a few heated bubbles away.

The good news is that they're both right, just not all the time or for the same things. So let's go over the benefits of heat and ice and why they each have their place is this world.

By far, there are more people in the pro-heat camp. Most would rather snuggle up to a heating pad than an ice pack any day. But aside from feeling good, what does it do? When you apply heat to an area of your body, you increase the blood flow, and blood does not travel alone. It brings with it vital nutrients and oxygen, two ingredients that promote healing in a big way. All this extra blood has another benefit, too. It not only brings good things to the site, it also picks up unwanted trash like lactic acid and other waste particles and clears them away.

Now let's look at ice. When an injury occurs, your body reacts and sends fluids rushing to the site, swelling the cells and causing inflammation. Inflammation is a good thing, because the extra fluids act as a natural splint and keep infection at bay in the case of an open wound. On the downside, too much extra fluid is what causes bruising and tissue damage. When you apply ice to the spot, it pushes away some of that extra fluid, reducing the swelling and relieving the pressure.

So does this mean that heat goes on an old injury and ice goes on a new one? It's a little trickier than that. Let's look at a sprained ankle as an example to help clear up the confusion. You injure your ankle and put ice on it for about twenty minutes several times a day until it looks more like your other one. A week later you trip over something, catching yourself in mid-fall. Although the fall didn't feel like a big deal, it could be enough for the inflammation process to start again. An injured joint can be touchy for quite a while. You can also have swollen tissue deeper in the body that may not be so obvious. This means that there's a third category of injuries to look out for: "new old."

To be on the safe side, keep your ice pack handy when you've done recent damage. Save the hot tub for when for an old football injury acts up. And pick up the phone when you're not sure and let your health-care professional make the call.

A Better Way to Lift

One of the main reasons folks come to our office is low back pain. All too often their story begins with lifting something without preparing their bodies to take the strain.

We like to divide these lifting problems into two different categories: correct body function and correct lifting principles. When muscular balance is lost, picking up something as light as a pen can cause the back to "slip out." This can happen as the person is bending over, before they even reach the object. This problem has nothing to do with the object itself and is called incorrect body function.

When the body is not balanced properly, it is susceptible to injury from ordinary lifting. An example of this is having very weak lower back muscles or worse, having one side of your lower back slightly weaker than the other. This can cause you to twist to the strong side as you stand up, leaving your back vulnerable to injury. A vertebra can be displaced, the disc between the vertebrae can begin to bulge, or a muscle or ligament can become irritated.

Muscle imbalance is pretty easy to observe once you know what to look for. There are usually significant postural deviations if an individual has had a muscular imbalance for a long time. Signs can include swayback, flatfeet, knock-knees, a protruding abdomen, or one hip higher than the other, to name a few.

Factors predisposing a lifting injury should be corrected before the injury occurs. If you suspect any postural deviations, you should consult your chiropractor. Proper management may include the adjustment of your spine, possibly followed by complementary alternative care.

On the other side of the pendulum, incorrect lifting involves a person who may have a healthy back but is using improper form. This is what we call a true lifting injury.

Simply broken down, correct lifting (or any type of ergonomic training) involves the use of postures and physical principles that leverage the body's strength to its best advantage. Lifting injuries often occur while in a hurry. When asked, folks often remember wondering whether they should attempt to lift something alone just before they hurt themselves. Accidents are not always avoidable, but here are some commonsense tips to help you keep injuries to a minimum:

1. Always lift in a vertical direction.

2. When lifting anything from a table, bring it as close to the edge as possible before lifting.

3. Always keep the object you are lifting close to your body.

4. Have your muscles partially flexed (contracted) when lifting an object.

5. Never try to lift a heavy object by yourself.

6. Visualize sticking your stomach out while lifting (this protects the discs in you low back).

7. Stand with your knees shoulder-length apart, slightly bent.

8. If your shoulders are facing in a different direction than your feet, you are twisting your back even before you lift. This is a vulnerable position for your back.

9. Always bend at the knees.

10. Use a dolly, wheelbarrow, or a bar for leverage whenever possible.

If you suspect that you've injured yourself by lifting something, it's best to see your chiropractor as soon as possible. In the meantime, try applying an ice pack to reduce the inflammation and minimize soreness. Ice should be used for about twenty minutes at a time. Remember always to follow correct technique when lifting and take care of yourself if you get injured.

Pre-Diabetes: A Warning Light

"If I'd only known, I would have done better."

A common thought after we're burdened with a preventable disease. With some, we don't need a crystal ball to predict because a simple blood test will suffice. *Type 2 diabetes* is not a condition that attacks overnight. It preys on the overweight and underactive, and it happens over time. A condition now labeled as pre-diabetes can be screened long before diabetes hits. The best part is that you can stop it with a combination of willpower and hard work. But before we look at the best methods to reverse a speeding train, let's get a better understanding of the disease itself.

An organ in your body called the *pancreas* makes *insulin*. I like to think of insulin as a ferry that transports people across a river to get to their jobs every day. In this case, the passengers are the sugars in your body that you get from food. One bank of the river is your bloodstream, and on the other side, we have all the cells in your body where the work gets done. Insulin takes sugar from your bloodstream and transports it to your cells. The ferry can also turn around and go the other way, back to your blood. After you eat a meal, you have a surplus of sugar in your blood; insulin takes the surplus to your cells, which use the sugar as fuel to get the work done. After going for some time without a meal, the sugar in your blood runs low. Insulin steps in and takes some of the sugar out of your cells and ferries it back to your blood.

When someone has type 2 diabetes, he either doesn't have enough insulin (too few ferries) or his body doesn't respond to the insulin he has. (Ferries have sprung a leak) This can result in having really sugary blood. Since your blood travels throughout your body, every part of your body can be affected by this imbalance.

So how can you tell if your ferries (insulin) are up to snuff? Most of the signals your body gives you appear after you have diabetes. There is a screening test that involves giving a small blood sample and putting off breakfast that morning. This test in not usually covered by insurance but taking it is definitely worth the time, expense, and effort. You can ask for a diabetes test at any local hospital or clinic.

While it's a serious matter, there is no need to hit the panic button if you have pre-diabetes. You hold the controls here, because things can often turn around with diet and exercise. This doesn't mean that you need to lose enough weight to bounce a quarter off your abs. It means modest changes, like going for a walk every day or drinking water instead of Coke. So many overweight people are malnourished because the foods they eat are low in vitamins and minerals. By taking a multivitamin and eating a few more things from the garden, your body will be more satisfied.

At the end of the day, it's the quality of our health that gives us the freedom to enjoy life. Live well now and invest in the opportunity to enjoy good heath for a long and happy future.

Reflexes: When Your Body Works Without Your Brain

The trip to the doctor's office is a journey that is equal parts mystery and dread. The experience is filled with menacing needles, that charming, backless, paper gown, the scale waiting in the corner, assorted clamps, gauges, and, oh yes, those mysterious investigative tools. Like that hammer thing the doctor hits you with just under the kneecap: what is that all about?

Among the many tests the doctor performs is the one that checks your reflexes. A reflex is a sneeze, a blink, a yawn in the middle of a boring speech. It's an action or movement that takes place without senior management (your brain) getting involved. Without conscious thought, your body protects you and keeps your factory functioning: coughing to clear the windpipe of any tiny intruders, blinking to clean and protect the eye, yawning when it's time to clean house, getting rid of extra carbon dioxide and taking in fresh oxygen. If a stray object flies at you, your eyes will close, your body will tense, and your arms will come up in defense before your brain has had time to identify the threat.

To look a little closer at the role of reflex action, let's imagine that we're cooking up some spaghetti (organic, of course, with omega 3s, because our example should be healthy). The water boils over and splatters on our tender skin. A sensory nerve on our hand is alerted by the hot water. The message is relayed to the spinal cord. The spinal cord transfers the message to motor neurons in our arm, and we pull our arm away from the boiling water even before the message reaches the brain, letting the boss know about the assault on your hand. In other words, the body springs into action even before the brain tells it to.

Our reflexes also act like windows to our nervous system, letting us know that our systems are working and evolving as they should. Some reflexes we are born with and outgrow; others we have for life. When the doctor picks up his little hammer, she is making sure that our reflexes are functioning how and when they should. If the tap on the knee does not produce the proper "knee–jerk" reaction, your doctor recognizes this nonresponse as a signal that something isn't working as it should and takes a closer look.

Let's look at the grasp reflex as an example of evolving reflexes. Place your finger in the palm of an infant's hand, and those tiny fingers will spontaneously curl around your finger and hold it in a surprisingly firm grip. This is a totally normal reflex action that is expected in the first few months of life. However, this reflex action does not remain with us for long. When the infant is beyond three or four months of age, the same finger-gripping reaction could be an indication of a possible insult injury to the brain.

From infancy and throughout our lives, our checkups include many reflex tests. If the doctor sees the wrong response to any of them, he is on the alert, watching for other signs. "Doctor" is the Latin word for teacher. As everyone knows, the best teachers are those who are ready and willing to learn from their students.

3 Self-Help Remedies to Put in Your Bag of Tricks

When you feel crummy, what do you do? Take a pill? Make an appointment? Get out your sorriest voice to call in sick? Look for a rare herbal remedy? Whatever your methods might be, it's always nice to be able to add to your bag of tricks. It's even nicer when it's natural and you can do it yourself. While these quick fix tricks are no substitute for outside help, it never hurts to educate the number one member of your personal health-care team.

Sinus Trouble: You can almost divide the population into two groups: those who never have sinus issues and those who often feel stuffed. My quick fix is to "rock the vomer." Sitting in the center of your sinus cavity is your *vomer* bone. When you rock this bone back and forth, the fluid that is blocking your sinus cavity is set free. You can rock the vomer bone by applying alternating pressure, first at the point between your eyebrows with your finger and, second, by pressing your tongue up against the roof of your mouth. Before you begin, make sure to have tissues at hand.

Heartburn: When heartburn hits, most people know that it's best to sleep on an incline. But did you also know that sleeping on your left side can be a big help, too? Your *esophagus* is the tunnel that food runs down to get to your stomach. It sits centered in your body. But your stomach is located is a little off to the left, just below it. By lying on your left side, you have gravity working for you, helping you keep those burning stomach acids down.

Sore Throat: Whether you're suffering from an infection, allergies, or an injury, a sore throat is a sign of inflamed tissue. Add salt to warm water and gargle. The salt calms the inflamed tissue by pulling out the excess fluids. As the fluids leave, the inflammation goes away. This doesn't solve what is making you sick but can make it a bit more comfortable while you're getting well.

Are You Getting Your Beauty Sleep?

Are you getting the basic necessities in life? If your answer is, "Of course I am. I have food to eat, air to breathe, plenty of water to drink, and quality, uninterrupted sleep at night," you're well ahead of the game.

The same is not true for everyone. Far too many people fail to realize that enough quality, uninterrupted sleep is as vital to our health as clean air, nutritious food, and water and that the lack of it does a whole lot more than make us drowsy.

Have you ever been around a baby who missed his nap? He's fussy, has difficulty concentrating, and does not eat well. As adults, we need our sleep just as much, if not more. When we lose sleep, we are irritable, fatigued, and easily confused. We tend to lose our patience quicker and take longer to find the cheese in the mouse maze of life. Our immune system suffers as well. We become more susceptible to viruses lurking just around the corner, because the reparative hormones that are normally released during sleep don't get to do their work.

There are many stages to sleep. The one that has the greatest benefit is called *REM sleep*. REM stands for rapid eye movement: it's the stage you reach when you dream. During REM sleep, your muscles relax completely. Your breathing and heart rate become irregular, and your brain waves are much like those that occur when you're awake. Getting to this stage many times a night is very important, because this is your brain's time to sort and organize your memories. The challenge we set for ourselves when we don't get enough sleep is that we don't get to reach and return to the REM stage often enough.

So, how do you know if you're suffering from sleep deprivation? Is the snooze button on your alarm clock starting to wear out? On days when you don't use an alarm, do you sleep in much later? Do your eyes open in stages? Are you less than completely awake until you can see the bottom of your coffee cup? If you said yes to any of these, you're probably sleep deprived and your body deserves better.

If you have trouble falling asleep, it could be stress. We are sometimes too busy to work things out, and we worry about our problems at night. Another factor is age. Our bodies produce less and less growth hormone as we get older, a handy trigger that makes falling asleep and staying asleep so much easier. We still need sleep just as much as we did when we were younger; it's just harder to get.

So how can we improve the quality and quantity of sleep? Create a regular routine and go to bed around the same time. Get some exercise during the day to work off some of the stress. Get some natural sunlight. Take the TV out of the bedroom or, at the very least, make a conscious decision to spend some quiet time reflecting and relaxing with your thoughts before lights out.

If you're juggling a busy life, the last thing you need at the end of the day is more chatter, clutter, and noise. Remember: if you treat yourself well, everyone benefits.

Sleep Off Those Extra Pounds

When you dream, do you imagine yourself running around scraping off those extra calories? Wouldn't it be nice if we could just dream our way to a more balanced body?

The thing is, it just might be possible. While sleep won't ever replace a treadmill or self-control at the buffet, lack of sleep can actually increase our weight. Let's find out why.

Statistics show that people who get at least seven hours of sleep per night are more slender than their sleep-deprived counterparts. To be more specific, those who get fewer than five hours of sleep per night are proven to be 73 percent more likely to be overweight!

Why? Unless you raid the fridge during your sleep, more *sack* time means less *snack* time. We get our energy supplied through sleep and feel less need to eat. Sleep also affects our hormones. The ones that are thrown off balance when we lose sleep are *leptin* and *ghrelin*. Leptin tells your brain you're full, and ghrelin tells you when it's time to grab some grub. When leptin is behind the wheel, your body does not go looking for calories from new food: it happily burns the calories you've already got stored. When ghrelin is in control, your body stores the calories floating around as fat and, with fork in hand, prods you to take on more.

When you are sleeping, leptin levels increase while ghrelin levels decrease. The hormone that says you're full dominates. When you lose too much sleep, the cycle reverses. Your body works hard to build up fat stores for a long winter that never comes.

Why would the body do this? Our ancestors had long summer days with an abundance of food and long winter nights with little to snack on. In the summer, we could sleep less and eat more. In the cold, dark winter, we would snooze more and burn up those calories from the summer.

How do you know if your body is starved for a snooze? Do you fall asleep as soon as your head hits the pillow? That's usually a pretty clear sign. Fifteen minutes is a healthier time frame to drift into LaLa land. Except for very rare case, those who claim to need fewer than seven hours are usually kidding themselves. With the exception of the very young (who nap) and the very old (who also nap), most of us need at least seven straight hours.

Give your body a chance to renew. Sleep longer nights to enjoy better days.

Do You Snore?

"Me snore? Noooo! Well, maybe a little, but it's not really a problem."

Many of us sound like we're sawing logs at night, but unless it's keeping everyone in the neighborhood awake, we don't think much of it. This is a mistake. The fact is that there are a few things you should know about this behavior.

Chronic snoring can actually increase your chances of getting other conditions, so let's examine what snoring is, why people snore, and what can be done about it.

As you fall asleep, the muscles in the roof of your mouth, your tongue, and throat begin to relax. If they relax enough, depending on the position of your head, they can partially obstruct your airway. When this space shrinks, you have a smaller space for air to pass though. Your body needs the same amount of oxygen so you begin to breathe harder. Forced breathing can cause the tissue in your throat to vibrate. The harder you have to breathe, the more the tissue vibrates and the louder the snore.

Your air space can get crowded for a number of different reasons. The tissues in the back of your throat can get too thick, or your *uvula* (punching bag–looking thing hanging at the back of your throat) can become too long. These changes are usually associated with weight gain. The muscles can become too relaxed from alcohol consumption before bed—there's alcohol in a lot of cold and flu remedies, too. Sedatives like sleeping pills work the same way. Finally, your nose may not be doing its fair share of the work. A deviated septum, possibly from a broken nose, may be to blame.

What do you lose by snoring? Sleep, in both quality and quantity. If the occasional stray elbow doesn't nudge you out of REM, the noise you make can actually jolt you awake. There's the daytime drag that you experience after your body overworked itself to get enough air and missed out on those restorative zzzs. And for those long-term snorers, the oxygen deprivation has been proven to increase the risk of diabetes, heart failure, and stroke. We tend not think of oxygen because it's everywhere, but getting just a little less each night can hurt every cell in your body.

There are things you can do: Since obesity is the number-one cause of snoring, shedding a few pounds will mean that your whole body—including your throat—gets more toned. You can try sleeping on your side to prevent your tongue from rolling to the back of your mouth. Some people have had success with nose strips. Many have luck with steam inhalation, avoiding big meals before bed, and investing in a firm pillow.

Everyone is different, and what's important is finding what works for you and sticking with it.

Sleep well.

Chapter Four:
Diseases

Health is a state of complete physical, mental and social well-being, and not merely the absence of disease or infirmity.

~ World Health Organization, 1948

Wilson's Disease

When you think about the vitamins and nutrients we need to function, you may think of omega 3 fatty acids, B vitamins, calcium, and magnesium. Very few people think of copper. This nutrient is one of the body's unsung heroes and plays many roles, keeping our bones, nerves, and collagen healthy. *Collagen* is a valuable body protein that makes up more than 75 percent of our skin.

Normally, our bodies take the amount of copper needed from the foods we eat and send the rest packing. For those who can't get rid of the excess copper, a big problem can develop over the years called *Wilson's disease*.

The symptoms for Wilson's disease usually start in the liver, where the excess copper begins to build up. A person might experience pain in the abdomen and a yellowing of the skin and whites of the eyes. These symptoms are so similar to infectious hepatitis that a misdiagnosis is often made. Furthermore, no simple blood or genetic test can confirm this disease.

Wilson's disease does have one distinct signature, though. It comes in the form of a rusty brown ring around the cornea of your eye. This copper-colored ring is called the *Kayser-Fleischer* ring and is unique to Wilson's disease. This ring's not something obvious that a loved one will notice when gazing into your eyes. It's something your ophthalmologist will recognize. Once the nervous system is affected, tremors, speech problems, and changes in behavior may appear. In its latter stages, Wilson's disease can make your bones brittle and cause the kidneys to shut down. Without any treatment, Wilson's can be fatal.

The good news is that after treatment begins, most symptoms reverse as the excess copper leaves your body. This is for people who get diagnosed early; left until later, it can create scarring in the liver, which is irreversible.

The work we can do to eliminate the problem is in two parts: removing the excess copper in your system and not eating foods high in copper to begin with. To get rid of stored copper, a patient is given a *chelating agent* that binds to the metal and sends it on its way. In rare cases, if the liver is just too damaged, a transplant might be the only option.

Although it is impossible to avoid all foods with copper, someone with Wilson's needs to avoid eating liver, shellfish, avocados, and nuts, to name a few. Though Wilson's disease is pretty rare, cases of it are all too commonly misdiagnosed. When a disease affects you or someone close to you, it becomes all too familiar.

Diabetes

Did you know there are 18 million diabetics in this country and many more that are well on the road with a pre-diabetic condition known as impaired glucose tolerance? Ten percent of the population is affected with diabetes, making it the sixth-leading cause of death in the United States. Worse still is the fact that it's rapidly on the increase. Ninety-five percent of these diabetics have type 2, or "late-onset" diabetes, and amazingly, only half of these people are aware that they even have the disease. Diabetes is a major contributor to serious illnesses such as blindness, kidney disease, heart disease, obesity, and amputations due to nerve damage.

What makes diabetes so dangerous? Diabetes is a disorder in which the body does not properly utilize glucose, the sugar molecule that is the fuel for all of our cells. When we eat, the food is broken down by various digestive processes and enzymes. When it reaches the liver, it is converted into glucose and secreted into the bloodstream, which carries it to the individual cells throughout the body.

Insulin is a hormone produced in the pancreas that allows the glucose to go from the bloodstream into the cell. Insulin works like a key, opening the door to the cell and allowing the glucose to enter. If there isn't enough insulin or its action is blocked, glucose starts piling up in the blood and doesn't get to the cells where it's needed. Imagine what happens to a drink if you keep adding more and sugar: it eventually becomes thick. When glucose levels in the blood rise, it becomes difficult to push the thickened liquid through tiny capillaries no bigger than a hair. When cells don't get blood, they die.

Uncontrolled or ignored diabetes can result in serious complications including:

- heart disease
- kidney disease
- high blood pressure
- accelerated aging process
- blindness
- stroke
- nerve damage
- blood flow problems
- loss of feeling, particularly in the lower legs
- high-risk pregnancies
- coma
- death

The good news is that diabetes needn't be a sentence of death and disability; in most cases, it is 90 percent preventable with lifestyle modifications. Rather than using lifelong drug regimes, patients can be taught to modify their diet, exercise, and take supplements that work as well or better than drugs.

Type 2 diabetes is also known as late-onset diabetes because it is brought on over time. Like many of our modern diseases, we're killing ourselves with a fork, one bite at a time.

In the past, type 2 diabetes didn't develop until around the age of forty-five or so. Now, thanks to modern diets and the pace of life, it is developing at younger and younger ages, even in children.

What are some of the signs to watch out for? Some telltale signs of diabetes include:

- frequent urination
- excessive thirst
- extreme hunger
- unexplained weight loss
- increased fatigue
- irritability
- blurry vision
- frequent vaginal yeast infections in women

The best test for diagnosing diabetes is the eight-hour, fasting, blood-sugar test. Fasting blood-sugar ranges should be under 100, with optimal levels in the 80s. Often, elevated blood sugar is the only symptom of diabetes.

In most cases, 90 percent of diabetes is preventable with lifestyle modifications, including proper rest, exercise, and healthy diet. Making these changes will optimize insulin levels. Once levels are stabilized, it is common for the blood sugar to come back to normal levels.

Exercise works by increasing the sensitivity of the insulin receptors so the insulin that is present works much more effectively and the body does not need to produce as much. To gain these benefits certain threshold must be met, however. Most people don't exercise properly and consequently don't reap the benefits.

It's no secret that the Western diet increases the rate of diabetes as compared with "traditional" or ethnic diets. For most people with diabetes or pre-diabetes, the diet must be radically modified. Diet modification not only aids in normalizing blood sugar but also has the added benefit of increased energy, weight loss, and a generally improved outlook on life. Some easy first steps include stop drinking soda, watch trans-fats, and limit simple carbohydrates, that is, flour and sugar.

Studies indicate that women who drink more than one soda per day can increase their likelihood of developing type 2 diabetes by 85 percent over women who drink fewer than one per day. Eliminating soda from the diet is probably the easiest and most effective way to lower your risk and your blood sugar. Getting started today will likely lead to an increased quality of life on many different levels.

Breast Cancer

Cancer has taken so many of our brothers and sisters, aunts and uncles, moms and dads. It's no wonder it's a topic not talked about around the dinner table or any table. When it is discussed, usually in a whisper, what we always hear is that early detection is the key.

If hiding under the covers and pretending something is not out there is your usual health-care protocol, let's try something new. Let's discuss early detection and empower ourselves.

Cancer is uncontrolled growth. Cells in our body normally divide at a measured rate. Cancerous cells divide very quickly, robbing the body of the energy it needs to do other tasks. This is why some people have unexplained weight loss.

With cancer, it's not just the size of the tumor that's important. We also have to ask, is there just one tumor or more? Has the tumor remained encapsulated in one group of tissues or has it moved? Is it using your blood or lymph system as transportation?

Breast cancer is divided into stages. If you're going to have breast cancer, stage one is a good place to be. At this stage, the tumor is no larger than a peanut, measuring roughly 2 cm. In stage one, the cancer has not spread to your lymph nodes or out of your breast. Best yet, the five-year survival rate is about perfect: 100 percent. At stage two, the tumor is a bit larger and may have spread locally to the lymph nodes right under the armpit. Stage three is also known as regionally advanced cancer. Here, the cancer has spread to the lymph nodes under your arm and possibly by your collarbone. The last one is stage four, when it has spread to other organs in the body. Treatment at stage four mainly involves symptom relief; the five-year survival rate is about 20 percent.

There is a trend in the health-care community of "breast awareness" versus "breast exams," meaning that you should be aware of any new lumps. But there's more that you should know.

For years, mammograms have been the golden seal in the detection of breast cancer, and most organizations are still really comfortable recommending them. But did you know that breast thermography has been approved in the detection of breast cancer since 1982?

While mammography uses X-rays, thermography detects heat from a tumor. There are three reasons I feel that this heat-seeking technology will someday replace its dinosaur counterpart. First. no pancake breast, no squishing, which will lead to more women willing to get tested. Second, there is no radiation. Radiation is cumulative over the years, and it's better to avoid it when you can. Most important, a mammogram is an anatomical study, meaning someone is reading the X-ray looking for a tumor. Thermography is a physiological study, which means someone is looking for heat emitted by the breast. Cancer is uncontrolled growth that needs an increased blood supply, which shows up as heat on the screen.

Don't ever be afraid to discuss with your doctor what other options are available. Know that when it comes to your health, you are the one at the wheel, and ultimately, you're the one who has to live with the consequences.

If this article scared you, I hope the fear motivates you to take charge of your breast health.

Multiple Sclerosis: Many Scars

We all know about the small ways our body lets us know when it's out of tune; a cold, the flu, and headaches are clear signs that the body needs a little tune-up. We're always ready to discuss these minor setbacks and share our sympathies. Ironically, when the time comes to take a close look at a bigger concern, no one wants to hear about it. When the body goes way off course and terms like "managing this disease" come into play, it's not considered socially correct to share. The tragedy is that problems that take more than TLC and chicken soup need special attention rather than closed minds and doors, especially problems like multiple sclerosis.

Multiple sclerosis affects our central nervous system, meaning our brain and spinal cord. Our nervous system, just like the electric wires in your home, works at a lightning-fast pace. In a coordinated effort of movements, all the internal meters send messages back up to the big boss, your brain. Although all nerves work in the blink of an eye, some are equipped to work double time. To accomplish this extra speed, some of the nerves in our brain and cord are covered with a fatty protein called a *myelin sheath*. Just like the effect of putting wax on skis, this fatty protein helps speed up the delivery of messages to the brain. It also acts as a protective layer that stands between the nerves and unfriendly forces.

"Sclerosis" means to scar. When this disease strikes, the myelin sheath is attacked by our own immune system. How it happens is that our defense signals get mixed up, and our antibodies and white blood cell soldiers go on the attack. The battle wounds sustained are hardened patches on the sheath that can eventually eat away the sheath and attack the nerve itself. The sheath is resilient and can patch itself, but once the nerve is involved, permanent damage will set in.

Our brains are mapped out and each section serves a different function, so the symptoms of multiple sclerosis can be widely varied. Some people may first experience numbness in one section of the body; for others, it could be double vision; still others may notice trouble with balance and walking. While every case is unique, most sufferers notice times when their symptoms are prominent (called attacks), with periods in between that can be totally symptom free. As time goes by, the symptom-free periods usually become more and more scarce.

For those living with multiple sclerosis, a wait-and-see treatment plan is typically prescribed for those with infrequent attacks. Medications are also available for controlling symptoms. It is also essential to take a proactive approach, to circle the wagons and get the support you need. Heat can trigger symptoms, so a good air conditioner is a necessity. Hitting the gym regularly, eating whole organic foods, taking your vitamins, and getting your sleep can help keep you strong. Getting adjusted can also keep the chips on your side. Know that this is a complex disease, but don't let that knowledge give you a reason to just roll over and let it control your life.

Multiple sclerosis is a serious disease that can assume many faces. Don't be afraid to ask questions or to reach out. A hug can pack as much punch as any manmade remedy.

Chapter Five:
Viruses & Allergies

Sickness comes on horseback but departs on foot.

~Dutch Proverb

Along Came a Virus

It moves in uninvited and soon takes over. It uses your resources to further its survival. It can stay in a quiet stage for years and wake up with a bang. No, this is not your adult child moving back home: it's a virus.

The term "virus" takes in everything from the common cold at the office that keeps the Kleenex box making the rounds all the way to HIV and hepatitis. Without getting too "sciency," let's dive into the gooey world of the virus and find out why this rabbit is such a tricky one to catch.

A virus is basically a piece of genetic material. Think of it as a composition of musical notes on paper. It has a plan—a melody—but it needs a willing player and an instrument to make the music come alive. In other words, viruses cannot do their dirty work alone. In order to be able to survive and breed, a virus needs to take up residence in another living cell. This is why viruses are considered to walk that fine line between living and nonliving beings.

Viruses are not picky when it comes to their choice of dwellings. There are virus varieties that can make themselves at home in plants, humans, animals, and in all types of cells. There are viruses that take up residence in the liver, like hepatitis, and viruses like the flu that prefer the lungs. There are also viruses that play leapfrog, jumping between species and creatures. When it comes to their human homes, viruses sneak in through the nose, mouth, or any breaks in the skin.

Can antibiotics help in the battle against a virus? To answer this question, it's best to think of this medicine as a selective poison. An antibiotic can halt the building of a cell wall or limit its ability to make sugar for energy. Next time the bacteria cell tries to reproduce, it dies in the attempt. Since a virus hitches a ride with our own cells, there is nothing we can attack without killing the host. With the virus effectively using our cells as a hostage, we can't get a good shot at it without doing some damage to ourselves. This is why the idea of taking antibiotics to fight a viral infection just doesn't add up.

Why does the body have so much trouble with certain viruses? With HIV and herpes, the virus sneaks in so quietly that we don't know it's there until the damage has been done. The virus mixes its genetic material with ours for several generations, breeding several new batches before symptoms start to appear. By the time the virus declares war on its host, the body has the cards stacked against it. Its natural defenses must retreat and let the uninvited guest do its worst.

How does your body ever get these squatters out? The good news is that your body is always cleaning house, taking care of many viruses that never get a chance to settle in before they're annihilated. Others, like the flu, enjoy a very short reign of terror until your immune system comes up with a strategy to take control again. The body uses weapons like heat in the form of fever and white blood cells to wipe out the invaders.

Appreciate what your body does for you. Try to return the favor.

Is It a Cold or Allergy?

It's happened again: you have a runny nose, you're coughing, and you just feel crummy. This usually happens around the same time every year, taking you down for the count and out of your routine. You're not really sure if you've picked up what's going around or if it's that beautiful bouquet of flowers sitting on your desk, so let's discuss the difference between the cold bug and the overreaction of your body's immune system, commonly called an *allergy*.

First, we'll look at what these two have in common: Both colds and allergies can give you a stuffy, runny, itchy nose. They can both come with a cough, and the fatigue can make you want to spend the day in bed. So what separates them?

General aches and pains in your body are unique to a cold. If you're feeling achy all over, rule out allergies. A fever sometimes accompanies a bad cold; this is your body doing its best to burn out the invading virus. An allergic reaction, on the other hand, never produces a fever. It does produce itchy eyes.

Timing is also important here. While a cold will last between two days and two weeks, allergies may last as long as you are exposed to the cause, sometimes moving in for a whole season.

If it's allergies you're suddenly getting that you never had before, you might wonder why your body is betraying you this way. In the age of disinfectants and antibacterial everything, it doesn't seem to make sense that airborne allergies have become so common. But the fact is that our immune system needs an occasional virus or bacteria to come our way. Without them, the immune system starts picking fights with harmless things; mold or pet dander suddenly takes on the appearance of a perceived enemy, and we pay the consequences.

Just as children exposed to the occasional germ—like those raised on farms—have fewer allergies, we do ourselves a favor to get out and about and toughen up our defenses. This doesn't mean that you need to open your home to colds and flu. To avoid getting a cold, washing your hands regularly with natural soap and making sure your kids wash theirs just makes sense.

But keeping your neighbor's germs away is only half the battle. I'm not a big football follower, but I am a fan of the saying, "The best defense is a good offense." Our offensive team is our immune system. If Sally decides to bring her date, Mr. Germ, to the holiday party, he can only get you sick if your immune system is low. Keep your fortress walls high with good food and plenty of slumber. Whether you take zinc or echinacea, get adjusted, or go for a walk to let go of stress, do whatever it takes to keep your immune system happy and you won't have to avoid the sickly to keep from getting sick. Of course, you need to take the obvious precautions: I wouldn't run up and give Sally a big hug, for instance, and I'll be saying thanks, but no if she offers me a sip of her drink.

In spite of its name, cold weather does not cause a cold. You may want to put on a sweater for comfort when the temperature drops, but don't do it thinking you'll banish colds if you do. We get sick more often in the winter because we gather together indoors, where it's nice and warm, breathing in everyone's germ-laden air.

Even with a great immune system, we can still get sick once in a while. When it happens, we need to take it as a reminder to slow down, to look after ourselves, to realize that the world will keep on turning if we take a day off every now and then and stay in bed.

When Is It Contagious?

So there you are at work, trying to have a somewhat productive workday. In walks a coworker who you'd normally befriend, but today this person has a serious case of the yucks: coughing and sneezing everywhere, leaving you with no place to hide. Wiping his nose with his hands and then touching everything, including the door handles you have to touch to escape, you feel trapped. You don't want to catch whatever bug he's spreading all over you. Just then, you hear him say, in a tiny, tepid voice, "Don't worry, I'm not contagious."

Could this be true? Can we really know when a bug has wings and when it has worn itself out? The facts often get confused with popular urban legends. Someone makes a confident statement, and with no one looking it up, it is quickly taken as fact. This is probably where the idea originated that we are most contagious before our symptoms appear. Many people believe that when it comes to spreading a cold or the flu, by the time we know we're sick the damage has already been done. This is not true.

Let back up and talk about the ways that a virus insinuates itself into your world. Whether it's from a slimy door handle, from a pen recently used by a sickly infant as a teething toy, or by getting sneezed or coughed on, after the virus has been spread to you it has an incubation period. During this honeymoon, though you have no symptoms, the virus is multiplying. War breaks out once the cells hosting the virus begin to die. By the time you begin to feel a tickle in your throat or realize that you've got a runny nose, the virus is running the show.

This is when your immune system goes on the attack. One technique the body uses is to burn out the intruder with a fever. At this point in time, you are an infectious nightmare, spreading the virus with every wheezing breath, juicy cough, gooey tissue, and sweaty palm.

What is the quarantine time frame? With a cold, we are most contagious during the first three to four days when symptoms have begun to appear. When it comes to the flu, adults are most contagious for up to a week, while kids can be contagious for up to two weeks.

It's always best, when in doubt, to ask your heath-care practitioner before heading out into the world when you're sick. When you cross paths with a sneezer, load up on your vitamin C, get plenty of rest, and do what you can to keep up a good defense.

Next time you get a cold, try to think positive. View it as a workout for your immune system.

Your Eyes: Not So Pretty in Pink

Your beautiful child wakes up and is having trouble opening his eyes. It's not from a late night of, "I'm thirsty, Mom," and other escape tactics from bed. He's got *pinkeye*, and when he does open his eyes, it's a sticky mess. As if you needed a reason to wash your hands before touching your eyes and face, pinkeye, or *conjunctivitis*, can be passed around, so let's get to the gooey center of the problem and try to clear things up.

What does pinkeye look like? It's called pinkeye because the clear layer of *conjunctiva* that covers and protects the exposed part of your eye and under your eyelid seems to turn pink. Conjunctiva is thin and transparent—kind of like clear plastic wrap. When this layer gets irritated and inflamed, the tiny blood vessels you normally can't see grow in size, mapping though the whites of your eyes to give off that pinkish hue.

The attack on our vanity is just the least of our worries. The eyes can feel as gritty as sandpaper, and rubbing them just adds fuel to the fire. The discharge turns into a paste while you're resting, leaving your eyes crusted together in the morning. You'll probably want to wear shades for several reasons: you look awful, infected eyes are often highly sensitive to light, and blurry vision can also be a part of the experience.

What causes pinkeye? We can blame a virus, bacteria, allergies, mascara, and/or other chemical visitors to the eye. Of these culprits, viruses take the lion's share of responsibility, followed by bacteria. How can you tell who the culprit was? If it was a virus, the discharge is usually watery. Bacterial pinkeye has a thicker, yellow-green discharge. (Oops, I hope you weren't eating while reading this article.)

Children are the most common mode of transportation when it comes to pinkeye. With everyone touching each other's things and then touching one's own face, it's no wonder. Conjunctivitis is very spreadable: you can be infectious for up to two weeks after symptoms appear.

Besides lots of hand-washing and staying home from school, treatment usually involves some type of eyedrops. The type will depend on what caused it to begin with. For those who like the home remedy route, the saline solution for soft contacts works as a disinfectant. Whatever you try, keep your health-care provider in the loop. An optometrist can sometimes get the clearest picture. If you're doing the right thing, symptoms should get better in just a day or two. After it's over, remember to wash your pillowcases and throw out any eye makeup you used.

Appreciate your vision and your health. Remember that whatever cure we feed it, it's your body that does the largest share of the healing.

Avoid the Flu Without the Shot

Are you one of those people who get the flu when the nights get cold and the kids come home with runny noses? If you've been watching the news and wonder about the effectiveness of flu shots, here are some tips:

Did you know that the shot only immunizes for the three worst predicted strains of the flu? Did you know that viruses mutate and change constantly? Did you know that the side effects of the flu vaccine are cough, runny nose, nasal congestion, chills, fever, headache, and muscle aches? Did you know that vaccinations actually weaken the immune system by introducing a live virus combined with table sugar, MGS, mercury, aluminum, and other toxins into the body?

Okay, enough of the negativity! Here are some great natural ways to keep the flu at bay:

Avoid sugar: Having a strong immune system is the key to fighting off viruses and bacteria, including the flu. Adding sugar to your diet immediately weakens the immune system because your body has to work so hard to process it. When you feel as if you're coming down with something, give the sugar a miss and add honey to that nice hot cup of tea instead! Keeping sugar out of your diet on a regular basis will improve your quality of life overall.

Get enough rest: The body does much of its healing when you sleep. When you get overtired, it has a tougher time fighting off illnesses. Regular sleep habits will ensure that you're strong enough to stay well.

Control and manage stress: Stress is a part of daily life for most of us, but when we become overwhelmed, it makes us ineffective and weakens our immune system. In fact, it has been estimated that as much as 90 percent of all disease and illness is stress related. What is important to realize is that the body does not differentiate between the good stress and the bad. Partying takes its toll, no matter how much fun you have, and all the sugar in party drinks and foods can undermine our ability to avoid getting sick.

Eat garlic regularly: Garlic delivers triple benefits because it is antiviral, antibacterial, and antifungal. Fresh garlic is one food that you should be eating every day.

Exercise: Exercising increases blood flow and stimulates lymph circulation throughout the body. White blood cells, which fight infection, depend on the circulation to get around. The more exercise we get, the more efficiently our circulatory system performs.

Wash your hands often: Washing your hands prevents the spread of germs from that first contact point to your eyes, nose, and mouth. Remember to use warm water and soap and give your hands a good scrub.

Get adjusted regularly: Keeping your nervous system clear of interference is an important step in maintaining a strong immune system.

Shingles: An Encore to Chicken Pox

If you're like most lucky kids, your mom probably took you to a chicken pox party as a child. After a little suffering, some serious itching, and a few bowls of chicken soup, you were granted lifelong immunity and chicken pox became a thing of the past. The kid who came to school with bumps all over his body, whose mom swore he was not sick, need not be feared.

Well, it turns out that the clear blue sky has a cloud: chicken pox has a sequel called shingles that can attack later on in life. One in ten adults will eventually get this viral infection that comes with less itchiness but a lot more pain.

We all know what chicken p[ox looks like: its fluid-filled blisters quickly blanket every square inch of skin. With shingles, these blisters are organized into concentrated patches that usually follow the skin over the path of a rib below. Because this is a viral infection of a nerve, the infection can follow the path of any nerve, even one on your face. This band of blisters is extremely sensitive (clothing rubbing up against it can be excruciating). Any combination of burning, tingling, itching, or numbness can come into play, and most patients feel the pain is out of proportion for the small area of skin involved. You can also run a fever, get chills, headaches, or an upset stomach.

Can you get shingles from someone else? No, not directly. Shingles is the leftover from your chicken pox episode. When it had run its course, your body did not get rid the entire virus. Later in life, when your immune system is low as a result of stress, other infections, poor diet, or medication, the virus can return in the form of shingles.

Until the shingles blisters have crusted over, someone with shingles can give someone else chicken pox. An adult who never had chicken pox but was vaccinated against it as a child is highly susceptible, because the immunity from the vaccination wears off, unlike those who came down with the real deal.

Shingles usually go away on their own in about three weeks, though some whose defenses are low may suffer for months. Treatment usually involves prescribing an antiviral medication and some form of pain management. Many natural heath-care providers can provide drug-free help. Keeping the area clean will keep the it from becoming infected. Stay away from heat, apply cool compresses, and keep the calamine lotion slathered on. Get plenty of rest and try to let go of the stress that may have triggered the outbreak in the first place.

The best treatment for shingles is not letting yourself get run down to the point where you are vulnerable in the first place. Though there still is a lot to be discovered about shingles, what we do know is that it strikes when your immune system is riding low. To join the nine-out-of-ten crowd that doesn't get shingles, you need to take care of yourself.

Chapter Six:
Pregnancy

Before you were conceived I wanted you.
Before you were born I loved you.
Before you were here an hour I would die for you.
This is the miracle of a Mother's love.

~Maureen Hawkins

My Baby Is Just Perfect

In the eyes of a new mom and proud papa, their baby comes into this world just perfect. To them, this newborn has soft baby skin, a beautiful round head, and not a blemish to be found. Strangers may notice imperfections and point them out, however, so we'd like to explain a few postbirth flaws that will soon fade away, leaving you with a happy, healthy bundle of joy.

Baby dandruff is known as *cradle cap*. It looks like yellow crusty scales on the baby's head, and it's caused be the rush of hormones that pass from mom to baby just before birth. It triggers the oil glands on the baby's scalp to go into overdrive, hanging onto the old skin so it can't naturally flake off. As a result, the baby looks like she's wearing a thin yellow cap. This condition goes away on its own, usually sometime before the baby turns one year old.

What about pimples? *Baby acne* is totally normal, and again, mom's hormones can be blamed for the outbreak. Don't bother with harsh soaps, just gently wash that tiny face with water. The skin will smooth out around the end of the first month and be blemish-free until puberty. At that point, it will be the child's hormones that are to blame.

Many newborns will have a few spots and dots, each one with a curious, quaint, or strange name. A brownish birthmark usually found on the lower back is known as a *Mongolian spot*; this is sometimes mistaken for a bruise. *Stork bites* are pink birthmarks found on the back on the head, where the stork would pick you up, of course. Pink marks found on the forehead or cheeks are called *angel kisses*. Tufts of extra blood vessels are called *hemangiomas*. There are two types of hemangiomas: strawberry ones that are bright red, squishy birthmarks and cavernous ones that are bluish in color.

Cone Heads: I couldn't leave this topic without bringing up cone heads because my son was born a cone head. Molding of a newborn's head into a cone shape is caused when the pressures of natural delivery make the soft bones in a baby's head overlap. Any fluid or blood collecting under the scalp can top off this look. Don't worry that your child will have to wear hats for the rest of his or her life: the baby's head will round out in a day or two.

These imperfections only appear in other people's babies, of course. Yours is just perfect.

Next to Everything, the Breast Is Best

Formula feeding is the longest-lasting, uncontrolled experiment lacking informed consent in the history of medicine. ~Frank Oski, M.D., retired editor, Journal of Pediatrics

Formula companies run a heck of a marketing program. They advertise in all the regular media, on television, in parenting magazines, and just about anywhere a pregnant woman might be. They are right there at the hospital when she gives birth in the form of free sample handouts.

In the '70s, formula companies were responsible to reducing the breastfeeding population to a meager 25 percent of new mothers, thanks to convenience and "optimal nutrition" claims. Sadly, breastfeeding had no fancy marketing team cheering for it, no one rooting for the home team.

It's time we take a closer look at the practice of breastfeeding, focusing on the long-term benefits for baby and mom.

Your baby's first immunization lies within your first feedings. Breast milk has antibodies and live immune cells to keep your baby healthy. Hoping to raise a future scientist or doctor? Better stick to breast milk. Special ingredients like D.H.A. and A.A. help breastfed babies have I.Q.s that average eight points higher than infants raised on formulas. As an added bonus, in these days of supersized everything, breastfed babies are less likely to turn into obese adults.

What's in it for mom? You benefit from a beautiful nursing relationship with your baby, of course, but that's just the beginning. Right after your baby is born, his suckling causes your body to release a hormone that helps the uterus return to its former size. And speaking of former sizes, breastfeeding burns between 200 to 500 calories (more than thirty laps in a pool) a day. That's reason enough to send out applications to become a wet nurse. There's also baby spacing, a decreased risk for some types of cancers, and the reduced stress from having a healthier baby.

And we can't leave out dad. He benefits in many ways, too, saving money otherwise spent on formulas and saving time and lost sleep otherwise spent mixing midnight formulas. And ask any dad if breastfed baby diapers are less offensive to change than the formula-fed models.

Mother Nature benefits from breast milk, too. Breast milk does not need to be transported or packaged. No other being has to be involved in the process of feeding our babies.

The last reason is trust. Trust that your body is superior to any factory in the nurturing of your baby. Trust that your body, which grew this beautiful baby, can continue to nurture your child after your bodies have separated. A nursing mom can nurse alone or with the support of her tribe. Her partner can take care of her so she can focus on her baby. Her mother and sisters provide gentle encouragement and guidance. And when she is nursing out in her community, a quiet smile can give her the confidence to keep nurturing our nation of tomorrow.

Pregnancy Changes Your Body

Pregnant women have been coming into our clinic in increasing numbers complaining of low back pain and acid reflux, among other things. The reason they're suddenly experiencing these ailments is that pregnancy changes everything!

The musculoskeletal system is the most affected during the last two trimesters. Over the course of a forty-week gestation, a mother's weight gain will ideally reach between twenty-five and thirty-five pounds. Because the bulk of this weight rides in the abdominal area, the woman's center of gravity shifts forward. To compensate, the natural curve of the spine—particularly in the lumbar/lower back region—becomes exaggerated, causing low back pain as the muscles cramp and the spinal misalignments and postural distortions trigger nerve pain. To help maintain balance, a woman usually develops a "duck" walk at this time.

Early in pregnancy, the pelvis begins to change in response to the release of estrogen and relaxin. These hormones also cause the ligaments, muscles, and cartilage to relax and soften, widening the pelvic joints. Although these hormones can affect any joint in the body, the *sacroiliac*—located right about where your back pockets are—and your *pubic synthesis*—where your hips meet in the front, often become the most unstable. While this increase in mobility will be a great benefit during labor, it can cause displacement issues throughout the pregnancy.

Digestive complaints are common as the pregnancy progresses, too. Because the uterus presses against the rectum and lower portion of the colon and elevated progesterone levels relax the muscles in the colon, constipation and diarrhea are common problems. Heartburn and gas are commonly caused when relaxation of the smooth muscle in the diaphragm occurs; hiatal hernias are frequent in the last trimester, caused by the pressure of the uterus squeezing the stomach.

A good massage can loosen the tight muscles in your lower back and improve venous return. Prenatal yoga exercises can help keep your body strong and your mind at peace. Chiropractic adjustments can correct misalignments, relieving pressure in the joints and interference of normal nerve energy, both essential for the development of a healthy baby and mother. Adjustments have also been helpful in minimizing digestive complaints. Most important, a good chiropractor can ensure that the pelvic bones are properly aligned, facilitating a quicker, easier delivery.

Pregnancy is a beautiful time to prepare for the new soul that has chosen you to enter into this life. Don't let these symptoms interfere with the joy you should be feeling at this time.

The Last Trimester

In the journey toward motherhood that is called pregnancy, the trip is neatly divided into three trimesters. The first three months are usually characterized by surprise and excitement. It is also the time when morning sickness is at its worst. The second trimester is when you start to show and everyone learns that you're pregnant.

Size and space can become an issue during the last trimester. The size of the growing belly will push the center of gravity forward. The curve of the lower back is exaggerated, and many experience back pain and pain in the area around the pubic bone. Getting this area adjusted by a chiropractor can relieve the pain in your back and make the delivery a better experience by lining up your hips to create the most space possible for the baby to squeeze through.

Space is on the baby's mind, too. Your body was built to grow a baby, and the baby will take all the space it needs. To make enough room, it pushes the mother's organs out of the way. The most noticeable one of these is the stomach. The stomach, and all its digestive juices, will get pushed and pressed up against the diaphragm, causing heartburn and gas. When the baby drops, toward the last days of the pregnancy, the heartburn disappears, but the added pressure on the bladder means many more trips to the bathroom for mom.

The last trimester is when the weight gain really adds up. Your baby grows the most during the last trimester, so the last thing you want to do at this time is go on a diet and start watching your caloric intake. Your body needs to burn fat to get the energy it needs for your growing baby. In addition, toxins are stored in fat, which means that they're released when you burn fat.

It's more important to consider how your weight is gained rather than how much you're putting on. Is it from increasing your portion intake of foods high in minerals and vitamins or are you a permanent resident at the all-you-can-eat dessert buffet? What you need to be eating are the kind of foods that will do your baby the most good.

During the third trimester another change begins to occur as a woman takes on the role of mother. With labor just around the corner, rational and irrational fears can bubble to the surface. During this emotional time, it's essential to find someone to talk to who truly understands what you're going through. Though you love him dearly, your partner may not always be the best choice when the person you really need is someone who has been through pregnancy herself a time or two.

Chapter Seven:
Hormones

The adrenal gland has a very peculiar way of slowing down when it has been overtaxed and overburdened. It fails in the manner of a large dying star, which gets brighter and brighter before it burns out.

~Karilee and Richard Shames

Menopause: The Second Half of Your Life

What does the woman who is going through menopause look like? She's somewhere in her forties or fifties, and she's probably standing in front of the fridge with the door open—not because she's deciding what to make for dinner, but because she's basking in all that blissful cold air. She gets sudden hot flashes that leave her drenched with sweat, and she may have dark circles under her eyes, thanks to those hot flashes that keep waking her up at night.

The reason she's experiencing these "personal summers" is that her hormones are out of whack. tThe cycle she once knew is changing, and her moods may be affected, too. Before menopause, a woman produces large quantities of the female hormone called *estrogen* and a little bit of the male hormone, *testosterone*. Every month, while she is ovulating, her hormone production levels go through a cycle. When a woman enters menopause, her production of estrogen dramatically drops, and as a result, the cyclic ebb and flow is forever changed.

Menopause is a natural process that all women go through. It is not an illness, though its major upheavals can make people think something is terribly wrong. It is a major change in life that can take years to complete. Whether you experience a few minor surprises or significant ones, the process takes some getting used to.

Technically, a woman has experienced menopause once twelve consecutive months have passed since her last period. Leading up to that time, her hormone levels can be all over the charts, causing mood swings, hot flashes, unpredictable bursts of energy, and bouts of fatigue. To make her experience even more difficult to understand and/or predict, her menopause will not necessarily resemble that of her mother, sisters, aunts or grandmother.

Dropping estrogen levels can make a woman's blood vessels expand rapidly, causing her skin temperature to rise. This is the familiar *hot flash* that begins with sweating and then, as the moisture evaporates, a chill that comes over her that can leave a woman feeling weak and slightly faint. When hot flashes occur while a woman is asleep, it's called a *night sweat.*

There is decreased fertility for a woman going into menopause, but until menses has completely stopped, it's better to be safe than surprised, so a word to the wise: never say "never."

There are also emotional challenges that many menopausal women deal with. Hormonal changes contribute to changes in mood and attitude, and many women struggle with depression and insecurity, believing that in losing their fertility, they are no longer useful or desirable.

When estrogen production drops, the male hormone testosterone can become the big kid on the block, even in the small amount a women's body produces. Thanks to its unchallenged presence, a woman's body begins to change: some women grow facial hair, many notice that their body fat moves from the hips and thighs to the belly, where men typically carry their fat reserves.

In most women, menopause comes on naturally. A *hysterectomy* can induce menopause before its time. If you do choose to get a hysterectomy, it's good to know that you can just get your uterus removed and leave your hormone-producing ovaries. In this case, you won't have periods and can't get pregnant, and you won't enter menopause early. If you get your ovaries removed, expect the early onset of menopause to follow. Either option is a big decision, so discuss it with your physician and invite him or her to explain your choices.

Because menopause is a natural phase in life, many women have turned to natural management solutions. There are many foods that naturally contain hormones that can help. Women in Japan and China, whose diets naturally include foods high in *phytoestrogens* (plant estrogens), navigate through menopause with far greater ease. These foods include soybeans, chickpeas, flaxseeds, and whole grains. Wild yams contain a substance that is very similar to *progesterone*. Though science is not sure why, they help ease menopausal symptoms, too.

To ease those hot flashes, you might ask your natural health-care provider about herbal remedies like *black cohosh*, a plant used by American Indians. You should ask about vitamins that support the female system as well. Even if you have a great diet, today's fruits and veggie don't always have the same nutrient values they used to.

There are also a number of simple, everyday things you can do. Try dressing in layers so that you have something to take off when the hot flashes occur. Try to find out what you may be eating or doing that could be triggers: are you eating spicy food, drinking caffeine, or working/sleeping in a warm room? Strengthen your *pelvic floor* by doing *kegel* exercises every day. This will help with urinary incontinence, which sometimes accompanies menopause, and works much better than crossing your legs every time you sneeze!

Ask yourself how you feel about menopause. Do you see it as a celebration of womanhood and wisdom, or do you see it as a time of separation from what you consider feminine? Do you see it as something that is controlling you, or do you see yourself guiding your vessel through this uncertain time? In large and small ways, our emotions color our experiences. Remember that menopause is neither a beginning nor an end but a transition. If you're going though it now, you need to remember that the changes you're experiencing and the challenges you face will not be with you forever. In other words, this new reality is not for life; it's for right now.

The Poorly Understood PMS

A female coworker discovers that her male coworker has borrowed her precious stapler again without asking. She staples a note to his coat telling him not to do it again. He thinks she has overreacted, and everyone jokes that her action is a sign of PMS.

PMS, or *premenstrual syndrome,* is one of the most poorly understood aliments out there. The prefix, "pre," is an indication that the symptoms occur before a woman's menstrual cycle begins. Women who exhibit erratic behaviors before their monthly periods suffer from this disorder, whose very existence is difficult to diagnose and/or prove.

Until the late '80s, PMS was considered a discomfort without any physiological explanations. Now, although it continues to be the butt of many jokes, at least it is recognized as a valid disorder. The difficulty is that you cannot get tested for PMS. No blood work can be done that can confirm or deny its existence. Declining production of estrogen and progesterone hormones before a women's period are suspected culprits in the cause of PMS, but this is not the whole story. Genetics, diet, and cultural aspects also play a role, which means that researchers looking for a root cause have their work cut out for them.

One thing everyone can agree on is that PMS symptoms are cyclic, in that there is at least one week after menstruation ends that is symptom free. (If your symptoms do not follow this pattern, PMS should be ruled out.) With about 150 symptoms attributed to the syndrome, no two women have quite the same experience. Some of the most common include weight gain, bloating, depression, and fatigue.

Although we may not know the exact cause of PMS, the good news is that we know how to ease the suffering by taking action and making simple changes. Stay away from salty foods that increase water retention and promote bloating. Take a multivitamin, especially one that supports the female hormonal system, to reduce PMS symptoms. Spend a few minutes at the gym several times a week to improve depression and reduce fatigue. For those who are thinking, *Who wants to work out with cramps so bad you can barely stand up straight?* prevention is the cure: if you start working out before the cramps start, they won't get so bad. You'll have yourself to thank, which will provide another reason to feel good about yourself.

With PMS, you need to look at things from a "glass half full" perspective. This condition is a reminder to take care of yourself: take a nap, do some deep-breathing exercises, honor yourself as a woman. You need to remember that that without these monthly fluctuations within the female body, life itself would not be possible.

Depression in the Happiest Time of Your Life

Your baby has arrived. Time to fall in love with the most precious one in your life. Your heart is being pumped up with a love that you never knew was missing. You couldn't be happier, right? So if you were feeling a little down, that would be really strange, right?

Well, actually, having a baby is an amazing, but intense, change in your life. It's so intense that, even when this tiny addition is a perfect wonder, it's pretty common to get depressed. It's also pretty common to be confused by such conflicting emotions.

The powers that be have divided postbaby sorrow into different levels of severity. First there are the *baby blues*. Up to 85 percent of new moms have this short-lived sadness and anxiety, and in about a week and a half, all is well again. Next is *postpartum depression*. About 10 percent of new mom's fall into this well. It can take as much as a year to climb out, because most days, they don't even feel like climbing out of bed. Finally, in very rare cases, a type of psychosis may form in which outside help is necessary.

One reason depression is difficult to overcome lands in the laps of those unhelpful souls who tell you it's "all in your head." The worst thing isn't their ignorance, which is considerable. No, the greatest harm they do is to make someone who is struggling with invisible demons begin to wonder if they might not be crazy as well.

Our thoughts and our stresses influence our overall well-being. Postpartum depression is caused by a number of changes in our hormones. Our estrogen and progesterone levels drop like a stone just after giving birth, much as they do just before a menstrual cycle, but on a larger scale. We also experience a drop in the hormones our thyroid gland produces. Blood production slows dramatically, and our metabolism slows down, too. All of this means that our physical bodies are running out of steam because we're not producing enough go-get-'em fuel.

On the emotional side, added to the sheer exhaustion from sleep deprivation is the feeling of identity loss. For nine months she was two: now she is a tired and worn out one. An unsatisfying birth can also come into play as well.

So what would a new mom be doing and feeling if she were depressed? She'd occasionally cry for no reason, she'd feel guilty for the smallest imperfection, she might go from singing the praises of motherhood one minute to feeling desperate because she can't keep up with it the next. She might also feel a sense of withdrawal from her circle of support.

To do a little preventive maintenance and stack the cards in your favor, get your tribe together before the baby arrives and work out an action plan. This eliminates the confusion that can happen when people stay away, thinking they shouldn't interfere or disturb. A good friend can get a meal list going of people who are willing to drop off food. Meals that come ready-made means one less thing for a frazzled new mom to worry about and a short visit to look forward to. Someone else can make a list of people who will stop by and clean house. You need to sleep when the baby sleeps and save the housecleaning for someone else. Getting dad involved is very important, even if he's only able to do the little things; a chance to shower while dad watches his baby can make a huge difference. And Dad, you can take care of mom during her recovery, making sure she eats, takes her vitamins, and gets her rest so that she can care for the baby.

If your condition is more serious than a case of the baby blues, don't shy away from outside help. Getting help does not make you weak. It's a sign that you're brave and strong enough to meet change head-on. Never in your life is your health more important than when you bring a baby into this world. Take care of your baby by tending to yourself.

Chapter Eight:
Energy Imbalances

The most sensitive members of the human and animal populations are much like the canaries in the mines. They are the first to show distress, often becoming ill for unknown reasons. They provide the distant early warning for us all.

~Karilee and Richard Shames,
Feeling Fat, Fuzzy, or Frazzled? *2005*

Help Yourself to More Energy

Most of us do things that lower our energy level. Constant repetition of activities detrimental to our health can become habits. Many times, energy can be improved simply by creating new habit patterns that are good for us.

Constant fatigue is often caused by a combination of body malfunction, which your doctor will correct, and poor health habits. Posture plays a major role in causing and relieving fatigue. When the shoulders are rolled forward and the body slouches, abdominal organs are depressed and the lungs cannot get enough oxygen. Poor oxygenation caused by something as simple as slouching in a chair or over a desk lowers brain and body functions. Alternatively, when your posture is good, your entire mental attitude improves: you look like you have a plan and somewhere to go.

Elimination of waste products is another important factor. When doing sedentary types of work (light housework or working at a desk), your systems don't work as efficiently in eliminating waste, and this can slow you down in more ways than one. You can cure this type of fatigue with a simple invisible exercise. Tighten your muscles throughout your entire body. Start with your feet and think of each area of your body as you tighten it until all the muscles are tense. Hold the muscles for five seconds then relax. Repeat the process a few times. This stimulates circulation throughout the body. Getting the blood back to the heart is dependent on using our muscles—one reason why people who are bedridden are at greater risk of forming blood clots. Follow this exercise with deep breathing to remove carbon dioxide and notice how much better you feel.

Deep breathing rebuilds the oxygen stores in the blood. When we become tired or depressed, our breathing becomes shallow and fatigue sets in. The stage is set for a vicious cycle to develop: the more fatigue, the shallower the breathing; the shallower the breathing, the more fatigue.

You've probably watched someone who is tired and depressed. They sit with chest sunk and shoulders rounded. Occasionally, there will be a big sigh. This is the body crying out for more oxygen. A yawn may be an involuntary effort by the body to get more oxygen as well.

When you are at low ebb, physically and emotionally, take the initiative: raise your chest to get a deep breath and then exhale, removing the stale air from your lungs. Continue to breathe deeply. Do this slowly. If you feel dizzy, you're breathing too fast. Develop the habit of using all of your lung capacity to enhance air intake. To learn more about proper breathing techniques, find a yoga teacher. Make sure you keep your energy running free by keeping your spine healthy and your nervous system clear. As the old Chinese proverb says, "You're only as old as your back."

Simple things you can to do to increase energy levels energy include drinking plenty of water and having a positive attitude. Liquids are essential for good energy levels: the more dehydrated an individual gets, the more fatigue sets in. Water is an essential ingredient in waste elimination and nerve function. As much as 75 percent of our body weight is water, which means that we should be drinking half our body weight in ounces every day to replenish what we use. Caffeinated drinks and alcohol don't count: a cup of coffee will actually pull about a cup of water *out* of your body, so try to drink that extra cup of water before you have your coffee fix.

When you don't take in enough fluids, you begin to experience symptoms of dehydration that can include fatigue, headaches, joint pain, muscle soreness, cramping, and thirst.

Attitude plays major role in fatigue as well. The person with a positive attitude, a plan, and a goal will enjoy a vitality that is not shared by those who trudge through their days because they feel they must. To put that spring back in your step, decide what you want out of life and how you plan to achieve it. A systematic approach increases the odds that you will reach your goal and provides no room for boredom, which nurtures fatigue.

Include time to rest and relax in your plan. A balance of work and play relieves the stress that we cope with in our lives. If you allow stress to build up and don't deal with your problems, you can make yourself physically ill.

As you follow your plan and reach your goals, you will be mastering time and relieving inner discord. You will not be the one who says, "I'm tired," when people ask, "How are you?"

Fatigue: Not Just the Winter Blues

Although there are many reasons people experience long bouts of fatigue, one of the most common is *anemia*, or poor blood quality. This may be caused by poor eating habits or by the digestive system's inability to absorb iron.

In general, if a person doesn't absorb enough iron, the blood won't have enough healthy red blood cells, which transport oxygen throughout the body. Iron at the center of each blood cell is what binds to the 02 molecules. It is also the reason that our blood is red.

If you've ever been at an altitude where you can feel the effects of oxygen deprivation, you know what it feels like to live without enough red blood cells. Because air is thinner at higher altitudes, it contains less oxygen. To cope, our body produces more red blood cells in order to transport as much oxygen as it can. Producing additional cells and getting the oxygen where it's needed takes time. Until it reaches its destination, a person may feel fatigued, sore muscles, and even headaches. Getting enough oxygen to the cells is the key to having enough energy.

There are also mechanical reasons for not getting enough oxygen in the blood. An example of this is when the rib cage is depressed from spinal curvature and imbalance of the muscles that activate breathing. To get a feel for this, do a little experiment. Take a seat and let yourself really slouch with your spine curled into a big C. Now notice the way your breathing becomes shallow. Notice how tired you feel. Now sit up straight, with your shoulders back and your head held high. How do you feel? How has your breathing changed? Go back to slouching and notice the difference. It's almost impossible to take good, deep breaths when we're slouching and equally impossible not to when we sit up.

Our circulatory system is constantly changing to meet the demands placed on the body. If the portion of the nervous system that controls this function is not working properly, fatigue will result. This is why chiropractors pay close attention to the function of the nervous system. Improper nerve function is often at the root of many problems, including fatigue.

How many times have you had a meltdown and felt like a nap a few hours after eating? The nervous system and muscles depend on normal blood-sugar levels to work correctly. When the blood-sugar levels are down, fatigue and other symptoms occur. Eating candy or other sugary products only provide temporary relief from this condition; it is usually detrimental in the long run and may make the overall condition worse.

Often, hypoglycemia is a warning of worse things to come; it is now being called pre-diabetes. One quick trick is to go for a soda or a cup of coffee to combat the "blahs." Unfortunately, this habit actually robs energy from our battery stores. It's like running your radio and headlights without turning on the engine. Eventually, the battery goes dead. In the medical world, this is called *relative adrenal insufficiency*, and it is quite common.

Your adrenal glands, which make adrenalin, are the body's source for quick bursts of energy. Unfortunately, they don't hold up under constant stress. Besides being responsible for much fatigue, other symptoms from adrenal insufficiency may be dizziness when rising quickly or visual difficulty under bright lights.

Thyroid problems can also cause fatigue. If the adrenal glands are like a turbocharger, giving us bursts of energy when we need them, then the thyroid gland is like the engine at idle: if your engine is idling too slowly, it's tough to climb a hill or get up to normal speed.

When the body fails to absorb and use the nutrients from the foods we eat, we experience many of the same symptoms that come with imbalanced diets. Half the families in the United States do not eat properly, consuming foods of such poor nutritional value that they become malnourished. Unlike the starved figures we see from underdeveloped third world countries, many Americans are malnourished and fat, thanks to a diet that consists of empty, valueless calories. These people are constantly hungry and tired because their food choices do nothing to nourish them.

Good nutrition is an important component in the good health equation. Fad diets that boost energy have no place in fatigue management and may even be harmful in the long run.

There are many other physical reasons for fatigue, including low blood pressure, chronic infection, and various pathological processes that your physician will check for. The most important thing is to find the basic, underlying cause of your fatigue, because it makes people uncomfortable, unhappy, and unproductive.

Iron Deficiency Anemia

Iron is needed in every red blood cell in your body. It's what makes your red blood cells red. When our bodies don't get the iron they need, our red blood cells get smaller and lighter. Those scrawny substitutes make our face pale and zap away our energy. So let's look at *iron deficiency anemia* and work on pumping up these cells back to size.

What would someone with iron deficiency look like? She (it's most often a she) is pale because the blood underneath is also pale. Her red blood cells are feeling poorly, which means that they can't carry the same load of oxygen as their healthy counterparts, so she gets tired easily. Her hands and toes might be cold from the lack of warm blood that normally keeps them toasty. She might get headaches and have brittle nails. And she might have a funky craving for nonfood items like dirt. (That's right, dirt!)

There are three ways to become iron deficient: by not getting enough iron, by bleeding, and by quickly increasing in size. Who is at risk? Vegetarians who skip the dark leafy greens (I call them "pastatarians") run a high risk of not having enough iron on their plate.

[The difference between diet and nutrition: Diet is what you swallow. Nutrition is what your body absorbs.]

Those with *Crohn's* disease might eat a bunch of iron, but they're just not absorbing enough. Excessive menstruation is an obvious choice in the bleeding category, but problems like an ulcer or polyp can cause blood loss, too. And quickly increasing in size usually falls squarely on the shoulders of pregnant woman, though it sometimes happens along with a growth spurt.

If this all sounds too familiar, don't start eating iron supplements like candy. The first thing you need to do is get your blood tested. If you're not iron deficient and you start taking iron, you could swing hard the other way and have iron overload.

An iron supplement combined with vitamin C (helps your body absorb iron) is the road back to normal unless the cause is a polyp or some other type of internal bleeding, in which case surgery might be involved. Eating iron-rich foods like meat, eggs, and beans should be on the menu.

Iron deficiency can be easily taken care of, which is a good thing to know because it can become a big problem if it's ignored. Your heart has to work overtime to try to pick up the slack for those lazy red blood cells. For a pregnant woman, this could mean a premature birth or a low birth weight baby. In babies and children, iron deficiency can stunt growth, both physical and mental.

Know when to give your body what it needs, and you can have the energy to do what you want.

Let food be your medicine

- Hippocrates

SECTION THREE:
THE MAGNIFICENT MIRACLE

Every man is the builder of a temple, called his body, to the god
he worships, after a style purely his own, nor can he get off by
hammering marble instead. We are all sculptors and painters,
and our material is our own flesh and blood and bones.

~Henry David Thoreau

It's hard to remember how incredible we thought our bodies were at the very beginning. Watch an infant experiencing the wonder as she begins to discover her fingers and toes, and it's still a stretch for us to remember what it felt like to us. Sometimes it takes an illness or an accident to make us appreciate what we have when it's in working order. Other times, it takes a close call to show us how precious our body really is.

The articles in this section take us inside, offering an up close and personal look at the workings of the magnificent miracle that offers shelter and support to each one of us. How it functions is an exercise in teamwork that is second to none.

- Chapter 1 highlights the management component in systems
- Chapter 2 gives us an understanding of the engines that run everything: our organs
- Chapter 3 examines the packaging called skin
- Chapter 4 looks at the mechanical functions of the muscles
- Chapter 5 explores our internal communications processes known as nerves
- Chapter 6 shows us how each movement hinges on our joints
- Chapter 7 even focuses on bones, the equipment that keeps everything organized

Chapter One:
Systems

*Let the young know they will never find a more interesting,
more instructive book than the patient himself.*

~ Giorgio Baglivi

Blood Pressure: How Low Should It Go?

Moderation in all things

One can never have too much money, be too thin, or have blood pressure get too low, right?

Wrong. We live in a high-pressure world of excesses in which our blood pressure reflects our abundance. It's a world populated by people worrying about high blood pressure, going to great lengths to achieve low blood pressure without understanding the risks when the pendulum swings too far the other way. So let's take a look at our excesses and revisit the old adage, "Moderation in all things."

The questions we should be asking are these: Can the pressure that helps move our body's fluid get too weak? Has *high* blood pressure hogged the spotlight for so long that we think *low* blood pressure does not exist?

We'll begin at the beginning, with a general definition of "blood pressure," one of those terms that you hear so often you don't give it any deeper thought.

Let's think about a two-story house and the water that runs through its pipes as an example. It takes pressure to push the water uphill against the forces of gravity. Too much pressure, and the pipes are just about bursting at the seams with all that water searching for the weakest link to release its load. This is the risk for someone with high blood pressure: too much strain on the blood vessels can result in an *aneurysm*, also known as a ballooning blood vessel.

When there is not enough water pressure to maintain the water flow through the pipes in your house, you may find yourself holding the upstairs toilet handle a few seconds longer, your shower may run in dribbles, and it might take ages for the bathtub to fill. In much the same way, low blood pressure forces your heart to work harder to keep every cubbyhole in your body supplied with fresh blood.

Just like the two-story house, gravity favors what's closest to the ground. In your body, this means that your brain gets the short end of the stick. People with low blood pressure often feel dizzy after they stand up; concentration is difficult, and vision can become blurred; they can become tired more quickly because the body isn't getting all the oxygen it needs; the skin is pale and cool to the touch as it thirsts for more blood.

Taking your blood pressure reading doesn't necessarily give a definitive answer regarding low blood pressure. While any number over 120/80 is considered high, or at least headed in the wrong direction, low blood pressure is diagnosed more often when someone has symptoms. (By the way, it's pretty common for an athlete to have healthy, nonsymptomatic low blood pressure.)

If your body is sending signals that sound like your blood pressure is too low, you need to see your health-care practitioner to find out why.

Certain medications, an overactive thyroid, even a heart problem could be the reason. But so can simple dehydration, which means that the solution may very easily come in a few extra glasses of water. After all the serious causes have been ruled out, get out your saltshaker. A *little* dash on your food can help your body retain water and get your body running like the well-oiled machine that it is.

As in all things to do with health and happiness, balance rules the day.

Hernias: A Break on Through to the Other Side

The body is an organized creature of habit with many chores to do. There is food to digest, new blood to be made, old blood to be destroyed, and general repairs and maintenance to monitor. For this machine of ours to run efficiently, every puzzle piece is given a job to do and a secure place to do it in. When one of these pieces feels squeezed from overcrowding and finds a weak spot in its retaining walls, it pushes through that weak spot and expands its territory. When this happens, a *hernia* is born. The body's routine is disrupted when a hernia takes up space intended for some other function. Productivity levels drop, and it becomes a priority to send the hernia back where it belongs.

Do people simply wake up one morning with huge hernia? Not likely. Most of the time, hernias start out as a soft lump under the skin; they're usually no bigger than the size of a marble and they're pretty painless. As hernias grow, they are usually divided into two categories: the ones you can push back to be flush with your skin and the ones that are rigid and stubbornly stick out. The stubborn ones are termed "incarcerated."

The problem with having bits and pieces squeezing through narrow openings is that the blood supply can get pinched off. When this happens, the hernia can quickly blow up like a water balloon. Without fresh blood, the sac begins to die. You can expect some pain and tenderness if it gets this far, and be prepared to go under the knife. Luckily, in most hernia surgeries, recovery is usually quick and complete.

Where can hernias occur? Let's take a roll call:

- *Umbilical* hernias are ones that babies are born with and are found around the belly button.

- An *inguinal* hernia happens right along the crease where your legs and belly meet. This is a weak spot for men. In the womb, the testes form in the abdomen and travel across this track to get to the scrotum; this path sometimes leaves men open to a hernia caused when part of their intestines loop out into their groin.

- A *scrotal* hernia usually begins as an inguinal hernia, but then the intestinal train moves down into the scrotum.

- I like to think of the *femoral* hernia as the female hernia, because it's the one most common in women. It rides right along the groin, too.

- *Incisional* hernias are blown-out scars of surgery.

- Finally, there is the *hiatal* hernia, which occurs when part of your stomach slips into your chest cavity though an opening in your diaphragm.

To keep your insides where they belong, you need to avoid lifting heavy loads. Any strain can make an old hernia grow or form a brand new one. If you find yourself wondering if you should be lifting something on your own, pay attention! Your brain is talking to you! If you're told to take it easy after a surgery, kick your feet up and follow those relaxing orders.

When a hernia forms, it's the body trying to release some pressure. Give it a hand. Try to relax.

The Lymphatic System: Your Body's Filter

When was the last time you thought about the lymphatic system? Maybe you felt some swollen spots on the sides of your throat the last time you felt sick. Maybe you remember your doctor checking them during your last exam.

As with most of our hardworking body parts, unless something is wrong, we tend to ignore them. And your lymphatic system is definitely hardworking. On most days, its work is a thankless job, so let's take a moment to honor this crucial system and learn more about its role.

The *lymphatic system* acts like the body's water treatment and filtration plant, keeping fluid levels in balance, filtering germs and flushing them out. *Lymph* is blood plasma. It contains water and nutrients, everything that makes up blood, minus the red and white blood cells. Lymph travels to the cells in your body, bathing your cell with nutrients. When it leaves your cells, it takes away wastes that can include bacteria, viruses, fungi, and old blood cells.

Arteries are like multilane highways that have lanes in which cells, nutrients, fluid, and oxygen travel. Veins are one-lane access roads that take the used blood back to the heart. Lymph fluid wanders through the body, visiting out-of-the-way places on the equivalent of narrow, winding country roads. The lymph fluid is drained into your lymph nodes through silk-like *capillaries*.

The lymphatic system wouldn't work without the *spleen*. The spleen recycles worn-out blood cells and fights foreign invaders. It is located on your left side, just under your rib cage, and if you can't feel it, that's a good sign. When the body is battling an invader—like mononucleosis, for example—your spleen can triple in size.

Healthy lymph nodes can grow to be the size of a grape. Most are found in clusters around the neck, armpits, and groin. They act like the air filter in your car, trapping all the pollution built up in your system. As the fluid passes through the nodes, it gets cleaned here. The clean fluid goes back to your bloodstream to do another flushing and cleaning cycle, while the nodes work on destroying the germs. The more waste it has to work on, the larger the lymph node gets. When you get the flu, your lymph nodes are working overtime and you can feel it.

The next time you start to feel a little under the weather and notice a swollen lymph node, be grateful that your body is hard at work and send a thank you to your lymphatic system.

The Thyroid Gland: Got a Lump in Your Throat?

Have you ever seen someone with a grapefruit-size mass bulging off the side of his throat? More than likely, it was an enlarged thyroid gland commonly known as a *goiter.* The thyroid is made up of two lobes, one on each side of the windpipe, just under your Adam's apple. It looks kind of like a butterfly from the front.

To understand what the thyroid does, it's important to understand the role of the *endocrine system* in general. This system is made up of a group of glands that includes the thyroid, adrenals, ovaries/testes, and pituitary glands. This group secretes chemical compounds into the body to control various functions, from your metabolism to your sex drive to how you handle stress. These chemical compounds are known variously as hormones, internal secretions, and chemical messengers.

The endocrine and nervous systems are closely intertwined. The nervous system controls the glands of the endocrine system, and the glands influence nerve control of body functions.

The thyroid gland is stimulated by the *pituitary* gland, a pea-sized gland located in the center of the brain. The thyroid gland produces a hormone called *thyroxine*, which stimulates metabolic functions and promotes growth. The thyroid also controls a portion of the adrenal glands, which in turn, regulates our response to stress.

Hypothyroidism: Running on Empty

Our metabolism is the rate at which our body builds up and tears down; in other words, it's the speed at which the body lives. When your thyroid isn't functioning properly, the first symptoms that develop are caused by metabolic change.

In *hypothyroidism*, the engine is running so slowly that a primary symptom is fatigue. No matter how much rest you get, you're still tired. Everything feels like an uphill battle, and virtually everything you eat turns to fat.

*Hypo*thyroidism means that the thyroid is underproducing its hormones, and this leads to lowered metabolic activity. Fatigue manifests as extreme sluggishness, decreased heart rate and blood pressure, and weight gain. The individual may feel constipated, mentally exhausted, and emotionally depressed—crying easily and often under the slightest pressure. In women, these symptoms can be further aggravated during menstrual cycles and can also include a feeling of fullness. There can be bloating throughout the body, including swelling of the face.

Since the thyroid hormone thyroxine increases protein that is used as a major building block in tissue growth, depleted levels of thyroxine cause people's fingernails to become brittle; their hair is thin and grow slowly; and they have dry, scaly skin. Internal tissues suffer similarly, and as a result, the body underperforms in general.

Hyperthyroidism: Put the Pedal to the Metal

*Hyper*thyroidism occurs when the engine idles too fast and we feel like we're on a treadmill. Symptoms can include nervousness, inability to sleep, and increased heart and cardiac output. There may be thin skin, fine features, and poor balance when standing on one leg. The individual may have an increased appetite, decreased weight, and erratic, flighty behavior.

There are several methods used to examine the thyroid; each has advantages and disadvantages. Checking hormone levels is a tricky business because they are always fluctuating up and down. Blood tests are commonly used but are often inaccurate, because different medications and nutritional supplements can distort the results.

Other tests can include checking the basal metabolic rate as well as the reflex speed of the Achilles tendon. Applied kinesiology tests the thyroid by using muscle tests to evaluate different energy patterns within the body.

Treatments are varied as well. While natural and artificial thyroid hormones can help balance the production of thyroxine, getting the dosage right is a challenge. As we've said, hormone levels are in a constant state of flux, and there can be repercussions that are difficult to predict.

The best approach is to return the thyroid to normal function by improving the body's energy patterns and supporting the thyroid nutritionally with food supplements. The body naturally regulates thyroxine distribution levels as needed. Medication takes away this control, interfering with the delicate interplay between the various glands and systems.

Remember, review periodically to determine the effects of treatment.

When Your Veins Get Twisted

Varicose veins are gnarled, enlarged veins affecting about half of all American adults. They feel stiff and rope-like to the touch. The word "varicose" comes from the Latin root, *varix*, which means twisted. Although most cases don't require medical treatment, most people would agree that they don't like the way they look or feel.

Varicose veins can usually be spotted in the lower legs. This is caused by the gravitational pressure that standing exerts on the legs. Your heart pumps blood to supply oxygen and nutrients to all parts of your body. Arteries carry blood from the heart toward the various extremities; veins carry the used blood back to the heart. Every time you tense the muscles around the veins, this helps push the blood back to the heart. When you stand still for extended periods of time, the muscles don't get to do their work, and the veins are unable to push the blood. One-way valves are used to push the blood to the heart but cannot do their job if the blood doesn't move. If the valves stay open, the blood pools and the veins become twisted, or varicose. Without adequate nutrition pumped to the surrounding tissue, the legs feel heavy, tired, and tight.

To avoid getting varicose veins, avoid standing still for long periods of time. If your job requires you to stand, try flexing the muscles in your legs often. It works just as well as walking.

Pregnancy increases venous pressure, so remember to relax with your feet up. A diet high in fiber is one of the most important ways to treat or prevent varicose veins. When you don't get enough fiber, your stools tend to be smaller and harder. This can make them more difficult to pass. Straining increases the pressure in the abdomen. This obstructs the flow of blood up the legs. Over time, this can weaken the vein wall and cause varicose veins or hemorrhoids. This is why people who consume high-fiber diets and remain active seldom have varicose veins.

For those who have varicose veins, elastic compression stockings are sometimes recommended, though they can be quite uncomfortable and difficult to put on and take off. Medical treatment for larger varicose veins includes stripping, or *sclerotherapy*. This process causes the vein to seal shut, stop transporting blood, and then fade.

There are plenty of options once you get varicose veins, but prevention is the best route to take. Keep those legs moving and be sure to get your fiber.

The Best Offense is a Good Defense

We've all heard the saying that the best offense is a good defense. That is, by not letting the other team score many points, we don't need to score many points to win. The same is true with our bodies when it comes to our health. If we keep our immune (defense) system running at a high level, we reduce the chances of catching something found in the outside environment.

Imagine this familiar scene. There's a small office space in a building with ten cubicles, one for each of ten workers. One of the workers comes to work coughing and sneezing. The next day, two other workers call in sick. What about the remaining workers who managed to stay healthy? Did they not breathe in the same pathogens? Of course they did. Were they not exposed to the same threat? Of course they were. The reason they were not affected is that their immune systems were in peak condition, working hard to protect them.

One of the reasons some people catch every virus that crosses their path and others do not is that our immune systems function at different levels. The immune system provides a first line of defense against unfriendly microorganisms. The thymus, parotid, lymph nodes, spleen, bone marrow, and tonsils play essential roles in the body's immune system. In addition, our antibodies retain long-term memories of all invaders they have faced. This explains why people only get the mumps or chicken pox once.

No pill or potion can ever come close to our bodies' amazing ability to fight off the constant flow of pathogens trying to invade us. So why does it occasionally fail? Why are we sometimes the one to catch the bug passed around at work? The problem often lies with us, when we fail to support our immune system and keep it strong. When we constantly overload our systems with immune-depressing substances such as antibiotics, cortisone, and antacids that destroy vital enzymes; when we eat foods packed with pesticides and preservatives that get lodged in our cells; when the body gets to the point where it can't distinguish harmful cells from healthy ones anymore, it either fights everything or gives up fighting period.

So, how can you enhance your immune system? Hands down, a change in diet is the most important first step. Removing refined sugar from our diet is essential. All forms of refined sugar can interfere with the white blood cells' ability to kill unfriendly bacteria, and when we eat within the guidelines of the standard American diet (aptly shortened to S.A.D.), we consume more sugar per capita than any other nation. Eliminating dietary food allergies is another big win. Many adults are allergic to wheat, corn, and/or milk and don't even know it. Identifying allergies has been more helpful in resolving ear infections than conventional treatments with antibiotics.

Once you've assessed your diet, consider other helpful changes. Exercise can increase natural killer T-cell activity, which helps prevent and fight infection. Stress is a major immune suppressant that increases cortisol levels. The next time someone suggests that your weekly relaxing massage is a luxury, you can tell them it's vital for maintaining your immune system. Regular chiropractic adjustments also keep your nervous system functioning efficiently, and your nervous system directs the immune system, so keeping your spine in line does a whole lot more than just improve posture. We use nutritional supplements to boost the immune system as well.

Those are a few suggestions to help you map out your journey to healthier living. Rebuilding your immune system takes time and commitment. The hard work is worth it, and besides, it's much more fun to work at staying healthy than struggling to regain your health.

Indigestion: One Big Problem with Many Causes
Part One: What the Big Deal Is and
How Chiropractic Can Help

Have you ever wondered why you are encouraged to "follow our gut feeling" or why we get "butterflies" when we are nervous? Are these just sayings, or is there more to it?

Science is beginning to acknowledge a truth that holistic doctors have known for years: the gut is much more than a highway delivering nutrients that keep us alive and well. It also acts as a "second brain." In his book *The Maker's Diet*, Jordan Rubin, N.M.D., Ph.D., writes that 100 million nerve cells are located in the gut (about the same number as are found in the spinal cord) and that nearly every substance that regulates and controls the brain can be found in the gut as well. Clearly, the health of the gut is vital to the overall health of the body, and this healthy state includes our emotional well-being.

Our digestive system begins to go to work after we have chewed and swallowed our food. Acting like a churn, adding enzymes and an acidic environment, it breaks down the food, preparing it for the small intestine. Once it reaches the small intestine, most of the nutrition and water is absorbed, leaving the rest to be passed through a one-way valve into the large intestine, where it is stored until it can be moved out as waste.

This simple summary of our digestive process tells us nothing about the complex, balanced ecosystem where there are more nonhuman than human cells hard at work. These nonhuman cells are the natural *flora*, consisting of billions of beneficial microorganisms that live in our digestive tract. Approximately four pounds of these friendly bacteria feed on waste, fungi, yeast, and harmful bacteria while they contribute to the development of a healthy immune system that prevents allergies and mal-absorption problems. When intestinal problems occur, the most common cause is a shortage of these friendly bacteria.

Reasons for these shortages can include diets that are high in sugar and refined carbohydrates, hurrying through meals, and overuse of antibiotics. We directly consume 5 million pounds of antibiotics every year. In addition, there is indirect consumption. Some 25 million pounds of antibiotics are introduced into the foods that are consumed by the animals we eat. While they promote weight gain and reduce infection in animals, these supplements kill our normal intestinal bacteria when we eat meat.

Along with proper diet, rest, exercise, and taking time to promote our mental/spiritual well-being, visiting a chiropractor is an important step in maintaining a balanced, healthy digestive system and quality of life. As chiropractors, we're committed to restoring the integrity of your nervous system and its 100 million nerve cells with the use of gentle spinal adjustments and soft-tissue manipulation. We also use advanced muscle-testing techniques to determine if any nutritional support is needed. Our goal is to help you maintain a healthy lifestyle that will add years to your life and life to your years.

Indigestion: Acid Reflux and Heartburn
Part Two: Your Diaphragm and the Hiatal Hernia

How many commercials offer instant relief for heartburn? With today's high-speed lifestyles and eating habits to match, it's no wonder people are looking for a quick fix. But heartburn is a symptom—a sign—that something isn't working right. Instead of taking a pill to mask or get rid of the symptom, it makes more sense to cure the cause itself.

What's going on when people experience frequent heartburn is a condition known as GERD, or *gastro-esophageal reflux disease.* Together with its first cousin, the hiatal hernia, it can be successfully treated in a safe and natural way.

Our problems often begin with the *diaphragm*, our main breathing muscle. This dome-shaped muscle sits between the chest and abdominal cavities and has several openings that allow the *esophagus* (food tube), blood vessels, and nerves to pass from the chest cavity into the abdominal cavity. Sometimes the opening around the esophagus enlarges and a portion of the stomach tries to go up through this opening into the chest cage. This condition is known as a hiatal hernia or the "great mimic," due to the numerous symptoms it can create. These symptoms may include heartburn, gas pain, stomach ulcer, or even an intensely sharp pain that simulates a heart attack. More commonly, a hiatal hernia will cause difficulty swallowing and a burning sensation as stomach acid backs up into the esophagus and throat.

Acting like a built-in valve between the esophagus and the stomach, the diaphragm is designed to prevent food from being regurgitated immediately after swallowing. It also keeps stomach acid from backing up into the esophagus. When stomach acid does get into the esophagus, there is a severe burning sensation called heartburn. Left untreated, chronic acid reflux can lead to the development of cancer of the esophagus. Taking antacids does not reduce the cancer risk. Rather than preventing or curing the underlying cause, antacids mask symptoms and often upset the stomach's natural pH level, causing it to produce even more harmful acids.

Preventative lifestyle changes may include not smoking, losing excess weight, avoiding lying down until two hours after eating, and eating smaller meals. Chiropractic care can help, too. By restoring normal diaphragm function and freeing the stomach, many individuals with acid reflux and/or hiatal hernias see immediate improvement. Nutritional support is often recommended to lessen spasm and pain, smooth inflamed tissue of the stomach lining and esophagus, and rebalance the flora of the gastric area.

While individuals with malfunctioning diaphragms, hiatal hernias, or acid reflux will not usually have all the symptoms we've described, some will be apparent. Because the diaphragm and digestive system are so important to good health, you should have yours checked as part of your regular chiropractic treatment.

Indigestion: Fat
Part Three: What's Your Liver and
Gallbladder Got to Do with It?

Do you know what the largest organ in the body is, by weight? I'll give you a hint: it's also the only organ that can regenerate itself if it is damaged. In fact, up to 25 percent of this organ can be removed and in a short time, it will grow back to its original size and shape.

Give up? It's the liver. The liver performs approximately five hundred functions that can be divided into two major groupings: scavenging and detoxification. The scavenging part happens when nutrients from the intestines enter the liver via the bloodstream. Like your local post office, the liver decides whether substances are to be sorted, packaged, shipped out, or held for later use. In detoxification, the liver combines toxic substances with other natural elements to convert them into less-harmful substances. Toxins include things like metabolic waste, insecticides, drugs, alcohol, and harmful chemicals that are neutralized for safe elimination from the body.

Of all the liver functions, one of the most important is the secretion of *bile*. Without bile we couldn't break down fats in the bloodstream. Not only would that mean no more trips to the all-you-can-eat rib shack, but it would also mean no vitamin A, D, E, or K, among others. Bile is so important that the body has a special place to store it so we'll have it when we need it. This storage area is called the *gallbladder*.

The gallbladder is a little bag that hangs just beside the liver, ready to squeeze bile into the bloodstream when digestion occurs. When all is well, we forget all about that cheeseburger after we swallow it. For people with gallbladder problems, it's quite a different story. Abdominal pain, bloating, gas, a headache, bad temper, and general sluggishness are the aftereffects of the fat hangover that occurs when fat backs up in the bloodstream if the gall bladder is inflamed or has gallstones in it. A gallbladder with gallstones is like a bag of marbles. It can do its job if the marbles are at the bottom of the bag, but if one clogs the opening or causes the opening to inflame, trouble begins.

About 20 million Americans have gallstones and gallbladder *cholecystitis* (acute gallbladder inflammation), and 75 percent of them are women. High-risk factors include poor diet, obesity, certain drugs, age, and yo-yo dieting. As with most diseases, it's much easier to prevent than to reverse. Fortunately, gallbladder disease can be effectively managed in many cases. Along with exercise, proper diet, and nutritional support, chiropractic adjustments can help restore proper function to the liver and gallbladder via the nervous system as well as relieve the organs themselves with manual manipulation. (Note: If your eyes turn yellow, seek medical attention immediately.)

I believe there is a natural intelligence that orchestrates the functions in our bodies and allows us to live this miracle called life. Chiropractors are trained to find and remove the interferences and obstructions, allowing the body to restore itself and achieve its fullest potential.

Indigestion: The Iliocecal Valve
Part Four: When Your Sewer Backs Up

Digestive problems affect people of all ages. Nearly everyone experiences one or more digestive disorders each month. For some, these disorders are occasional; for others, the trouble is chronic.

Digestion occurs in three phases. The first phase begins when we chew our food. While saliva is breaking down the food, the taste buds send messages to the stomach to begin secreting digestive acids. Phase two begins once the food enters the stomach. There, it's churned and broken down in acid with a pH level as low as one. To give you an idea how strong that is, if you were able to put your hand into your stomach, the acid would eat it down to the bone in no time. The third and final phase occurs when food leaves the stomach and enters the small intestine. There, enzymes break food to particles small enough to be absorbed through the intestinal walls to be used by the cells. What is left over is considered waste and is passed into the large intestine for temporary storage and elimination.

Between the small and large intestines there is a one-way valve called the *iliocecal valve*, which opens and closes like a door. It serves as a gate, keeping nutrient-rich food in the small intestine and allowing the waste to pass through to the large intestine once the body has taken what it wants. The problem arises when the iliocecal valve gets stuck open or closed.

A closed valve causes waste to remain too long in the small intestine. If the body absorbs it, your entire system can become toxic, because the body is literally eating its own feces. When your body is toxic, the weakest links in your systems, organs, and muscles are affected. All kinds of symptoms can arise, including, but not limited to: shoulder pain, sudden low back pain, dizziness, ringing in the ears, flulike symptoms, headache symptoms, dark circles under the eyes, nausea, faintness, symptoms mimicking IBS, sudden thirst, and bowel involvement.

One thing that most sufferers have in common is that symptoms usually improve after getting out of bed and moving around; they also intensify with inactivity.

A valve stuck open creates similar problems, because the waste doesn't stay in the large intestines where it belongs. With no gate to keep it down the line, it's like having your sewer back up, causing similar symptoms to those listed previously.

We check the iliocecal valve as part of a regular chiropractic visit. Because the valve functions as a reaction to the nerve that controls it, there are simple adjustments that can be done to help remedy the problem. Certain nutritional supplements are typically prescribed as well. Muscle testing allows us to ask the body questions directly, avoiding the confusion of trying to chase down and treat every symptom individually. The goal of chiropractic is to find the underlying cause of the problem, remove it, and then let the body heal naturally.

Breathe, Breathe in the Air

Man must breathe. From the first deep inhale of a newborn signaling its arrival to this life until the last exhale that comes with our departure, we must breathe. This most vital of functions continues automatically at around 3 seconds per cycle, 28,000 times per day, every day of our lives. Like the beat of our heart, the digestion of our food, and the flow of our nerves, breathing is controlled unconsciously so that we can go about our lives without having to worry about it.

Any two-year-old quickly discovers that they can hold their breath, and in doing so, they unlock one of the great secrets of life. The fact that we can control our breathing, making it both a conscious and an unconscious function, not only separates it from all other autonomic functions, it actually bridges the body and the mind. Due to its double nature, we gain the means for conscious participation in the most vital and universal function of our being.

Let me give you an example. We all know that when we get stressed out, our breathing becomes shallow and rapid; conversely, just as we're on the edge of sleep, our breathing is slow and deep. There is a direct tie between the quality of the breath and these states of being. Now, imagine that you're stressed, and you take control of your breath. You begin to breathe deep and slow breaths. Lo and behold, the stress starts to dissipate, and you begin to relax. That's a pretty nifty trick if you learn to use it, and it's just the tip of the iceberg. Many advanced religions and traditions, like yoga, have very sophisticated techniques regarding the use of breath.

Another important aspect of breathing is to get into the habit of breathing through the nose. Any yoga or track coach will tell you to do this, but why? When we breathe through our noses, we stimulate the olfactory nerve, which is a direct extension of the brain. In fact, the left and right nasal rhythm actually reflects the hemispheric activity of the brain.

Take a moment and notice which nostril is easier to breathe through. Right nostril dominance goes with the left hemisphere and vice versa. Next time your sinuses are clogged, notice which side is full and then check again in about twenty minutes. More than likely it will have switched sides. This reflects the same natural rhythm of the hemispheres of the brain.

The next time you feel stressed or fatigued, take ten deep inhales through the nostrils, hold for five seconds, and briskly exhale through the nostrils. This will usually strip the unwanted charges from the body and bring it to a state of balance and well-being.

The mouth breather is challenged by several problems. Perhaps the most common is when people hold their breath as soon as they are stressed. The slightest trauma, psychological or physical, causes an activation of the solar plexus, which produces an emotional stimuli and the holding of breath. This weakens our life energy at the moment when we need it most. Thus, the more our breath is freed up, the less the effect of the trauma.

As part of a regular chiropractic visit, we check the solar plexus using muscle testing and, when needed, a specific technique to release the solar plexus developed by Wilhelm Reich called *shock release*. Oftentimes, the patient notices an emotional release within the next day or two. By clearing the nervous system, the patient's breath becomes more full, clear, and deep.

Remember, the next time you feel stuck in any way, sit up straight, take a couple of deep breaths, and appreciate what an amazing miracle it is to be alive.

Chapter Two:
Organs

Man is an intelligence in servitude to his organs.

~Aldous Huxley

Appendicitis

The Egyptians called the *appendix* the "the worm of the intestines." Many of us have ours removed before trouble starts, and most people say it has no use in our body to start with. It's not often that we find something in our bodies that has no practical purpose, so let's take a closer look at the appendix and find out how it goes from being the wallflower at the party to a serious threat. We'll find out what causes the body to give it the pink slip known as *appendicitis*.

The appendix is about the size and shape of a finger. It's located below your belly button on the right side, between the small intestine and the colon. After food works its way through your stomach and small intestine, it goes to the colon. Since the appendix is a dead end, the colon is the only way out.

If the appendix is a dead end, what is it good for? The short answer is that no one is quite sure. Some argue that the appendix is a vestigial organ, meaning that whatever use it had is no longer required in modern man. Others point out that the appendix contains a great number of lymph channels and suggest that it could regulate the bacteria population in the gut. My feeling is that if we don't have its function figured out, it means that we have more work to do. Suggesting that the appendix has no purpose simply because we can't see it seems a little arrogant.

Appendicitis (remember that "itis" means that something is inflamed) usually begins with an obstruction (typically food waste or a fecal stone). This is felt as pain right around the belly button. The lining of the appendix secretes mucus, which becomes plugged up and has nowhere to go. Like a water balloon, this pouch gets filled up, and the aching pain moves over to your right lower abdomen. With appendicitis, you'll get something called *rebound tenderness*, meaning that if you press into the spot over the appendix, it will be pretty tender. Nausea, swelling, a low-grade fever, and constipation or diarrhea can also show up as the body goes into action, trying to eject the offending matter.

The whole build-up happens in less than a half a day, so timely action is definitely called for. Without a blood supply, the appendix will die (necrosis), and pressure can cause it to burst open (rupture). If it ruptures, this is a medical emergency. Surgical removal of the appendix is the way to go, and thanks to *laparoscopic surgery* involving minimal invasion techniques, the patient is left with just a tiny scar.

The good news is that you can keep this little "worm" safe from harm by following a diet that is high in natural (less-processed) fiber. While most of us Westerners think appendicitis is pretty common, there's no reason not to maintain a healthy appendix and digestive system to match.

There is a time for everything. With appendicitis, it's not the time to sit and wait it out.

Here's to You, Kidneys

What do we really know about our kidneys? They come in sets of two and make urine. Every now and then, we hear of someone donating one, which must mean that one kidney must be able to work on its own. But other than acting as collection stations for urine, what's the big deal?

The kidneys are about the size of a computer mouse. They sit in the back of the abdomen, on either side of the spine, usually just below the last rib. They are reddish brown and bean shaped. If you hear the term *renal*, know that it's your kidneys that are being discussed.

First and foremost, kidneys are filters. Like those paper cones in your coffeepot, your kidneys sift through water, ions, glucose, and small proteins, mining what it needs. It works to remove everything, from the toxins that got into your food to the medicine you took. Together, they can filter though about 180 liters each day. Considering that we only have seven to eight liters of blood in our bodies, they clearly don't mind repetitive work.

So how does the filtration process work? Let's say you indulge in a big tub of salty popcorn. The sodium makes its way through your digestive tract. In the intestines, it gets absorbed into your bloodstream. When the blood reaches your kidneys, they pull the extra salt—also known as an *electrolyte*—out of your system. Sodium is just one of the electrolytes it keeps in check.

What if you don't drink enough water? How do your kidneys know ahead of time to hold back the fluids it has? A gland in your brain figures out how much water you have to spare, based on the sodium concentration in your blood. If liquids need to be saved, an *antidiuretic* hormone is released, and the body reabsorbs water.

How do you know if your body is holding back? Check the color of your urine. If you are properly hydrated, it should be a very light yellow. In fact, the guideline is that if all is well, your urine should be as light as the color of straw. Any darker and it's time to hit the water cooler.

Kidneys don't stop at filtration. They also make their own hormones and do their part in balancing your blood pressure.

The more you learn how your body works, the more you'll respect and take of it.

When Your Kidneys Get Stoned

There are moments in life the memory keeps forever fresh. You never forget your wedding day, the first time you held your darling little baby, and, if you're unlucky, that time you passed a kidney stone.

The pain from passing these pebbles is hard to forget, so let's get to know about them and find out what we can do to avoid them. Kidney stones, which take up residence in the kidneys, are not bad tenants. It's when they decide to move out that the horror begins. When a stone breaks loose from the kidney, it travels down a tunnel called the *urethra* on its way to your bladder. This journey can be really painful, because the urethra is not designed to carry solid passengers.

What can it feel like? It's an intense, colicky pain that changes intensity every five to fifteen minutes. The pain follows the path of the stone, beginning in your back, just under your ribs, and traveling all the way down to where your bladder is. The sufferer may be nauseated and have the feeling that he has to urinate all the time. A fever is a sign that you also have an infection, which needs tending to. The reason you need to go and see a health-care professional is to make sure that the fever is not caused by a tearing of the urethra as the stone moves.

Most kidney stones are made up of calcium. We don't really understand why they happen, but dehydration, diet choices, lack of exercise, and certain medications all play a role.

How do we stay stone free? You should be passing at least 2.5 quarts of water a day. To do that, you have to drink 3.5 quarts of water each day: translation—you should drink fourteen glasses a day. The more you sweat, the more you should drink.

Why so much water? It dilutes everything you eat and cleanses the body. If you've already passed a kidney stone, you want to avoid eating organ meats, anchovies, chocolate (sorry), and berries. Many natural health-care professionals would recommend eating foods high in magnesium (like tofu or pumpkin seeds) and drinking natural cranberry juice.

When your body starts throwing up signals onto your radar, you have two choices: you can ignore them or seek out the cause. Pick the latter. When you discover the "what" and, hopefully, the "why," you can decide to ignore it, but at least your decision will be an educated one.

Long Live the Liver

The liver works hard, performing a thankless job. Second only to the skin when it comes to the size of its workload, the liver is a powerful organ. While it does most things right, things can and do occasionally go wrong. When the liver becomes bloated and inflamed, we called it *hepatitis*. When it scars up and scabs over, it becomes *cirrhosis*. Let's find out why these conditions occur and what we can do to prevent them from happening.

Your liver lives just under your rib cage, on the right side of your body. If you squint a little, you could say it's shaped like an ice cream cone, with the pointy side headed toward the midline of your body. The liver is the only organ that can regenerate itself; up to 80 percent of it can be removed in surgery, and within weeks, it will grow back. In Greek mythology, Prometheus was chained to a rock, where a vulture would peck out his liver and it would grow back overnight.

If spontaneous regeneration wasn't enough to impress you, the liver also works overtime doing hundred of tasks, many of which involve sorting everything that you drink, eat, and breathe. From the good stuff your body needs, the liver breaks up nutrients into usable by-products. It then sends them out to the rest of the body, hitching their ride on the bloodstream.

Your liver also sorts and metabolizes toxins so they can be safely flushed out of your system.

Toxins can be anything from alcohol to drugs. Your liver considers medication a drug; it doesn't care if it was prescribed. There are also the less-obvious suspects, like toxic pesticides and chemicals from aerosol sprays. Waste that will eventually leave through your urine it sends to your kidneys via the bloodstream. A stream of greenish fluid called bile carries the rest away. This goes straight to your digestive system and is taxied away with your feces.

The liver can multitask like a mother of three, acting as a storage locker for sugar, waiting for the body to request the extra energy. Its bile makes fat digestion possible. It makes the good cholesterol that is needed by every cell in our body. It even helps the immune system so your neighbor's germs don't come over for a visit.

Unfortunately, the liver is not indestructible. Before you lift up your next beer and say cheers, know that your liver can only handle so much. There are many toxins in the air and environment. Adding unnecessary toxins to your body can often be too much for this organ to handle. Modern society gives the liver plenty of reasons to stay busy, so you need to pay attention and give it a helping hand. Watching what you put on your skin and put in mouth can help your liver from pulling overtime. You can find other ways to detoxify your system so that your liver doesn't have to work alone. Sweating more—which means exercising more—is a good first step.

Be thankful for the parts that make up you. Do this while they are working as they should. Your appreciation and self-care won't go unnoticed.

Chapter Three:
Skin

I love the body. Flesh is so honest, and organs do not lie.

~Candea Core-Starke

Dermatitis

When springtime springs upon us, it's time to switch out the heavy pants and sweaters for something a little lighter. It's also time to pay attention to the skin that's been under wraps, especially if the itchy bits are red and swollen in spots.

Dermatitis, which also goes by the name *eczema*, is so common that we need to stop ignoring it and learn how to send it packing.

Our *derma* is our skin and any "itis" is an inflammation. So dermatitis is an inflammation of the skin. Your dermatitis may not look like your neighbor's, because there are many varieties to choose from. What they all have in common is redness, itching, swelling, and skin lesions that can be quite uncomfortable and not too pretty to look at. If ignored long enough, it can become *cellulitis*, a deeper infection whose red streaks under the skin will require medical attention.

Your skin acts as a barrier, keeping all your fluids inside and the rest of the world at bay. This wall of defense begins to crumble as the skin dries out—something that often happens when the skin is exposed to the harsh winter air. This leaves the gate open for irritants and allergens to break through. An irritant or allergen might be perfume, makeup, or chemicals from your dryer sheet rubbing off onto your clothes. Your body reacts by bringing extra blood, including those defensive white blood cells, to the irritated area. The extra blood makes the area red and puffy. You could also be eating something your body is sensitive to. As some of the toxins leave by way of the skin, red itchy areas are left in its tracks.

A good first step to prevent dry skin from becoming a problem is to moisturize. This helps seal the cracks in the barrier that your skin provides. For sufferers with inflamed skin, a good choice in moisturizers is a natural one with chamomile, which has anti-inflammatory properties in it.

Your skin also dries up if you're not getting enough water, so stay hydrated. And look at the chemicals you're putting on that part of your body. This could be a sign to change detergents or perfumed skin creams. There are many natural alternatives for everything on the market. As a general rule, unscented and dye-free products have fewer irritants. Once you get rid of what's bothering your skin, your body will thank you and let the healing begin.

Often the body gives us signs and signals. Be your own detective and become the best advocate for your health.

Fingernails: Ten Tiny Windows to Your Health

Some people put layers on them. Some adorn theirs with jewels and lather them in lotion. Most people let them go completely nude for everyone to see. Some keep them neat and clean, while others let them grow wild and free. Of course we're talking about fingernails here.

Besides being something to decorate, clean, cut, or maybe bite, they are windows to our health. They can become pitted, change colors, and even become detached, all of these changes giving clues that something's not right with your overall health.

Let's start with the color. White spots on your nails are usually signs of a vitamin or mineral deficiency. To get rid of these spots, increase the fruits and veggies and eat fewer processed foods. Your nails can take on a slightly greenish or yellow hue in a condition called *yellow nail syndrome*. This happens when the growth of your nails slows down due to a respiratory problem or from your fingers swelling. A bluish hue accompanied by trouble breathing is a sign of lack of oxygen; the blue color without trouble breathing is most likely exposure to a toxic chemical.

Shape and Contour: Pitted nails look like they have little potholes, a condition that usually accompanies *psoriasis*. Clubbed nails thicken and begin to curve around your fingertips, a sign of low oxygen levels in your blood.

A condition called *spoon nails* happens when the sides of the nails curve out and you can actually hold a drop of water in them. It's a sign of iron deficiency anemia. Splintered nails that were not caused by an accident and do not hurt could be a sign of a serious heart condition. You should get it checked out ASAP.

When your nails become more flexible than they used to be, this is usually a deficiency of calcium or protein. When your nail begins to separate from the finger bed, this could be a result of an injury, a drug reaction, psoriasis, thyroid disease, or a reaction to acrylic nails.

If you notice any change in your nails, be sure to get it checked out by a qualified individual. The cure might involve some vitamins, a homeopathic remedy, or more serious medical attention.

Be good to yourself. Your nails are more than decorative: they're windows to your health.

Know Your Moles

Summer is a wonderful time to enjoy plenty of fresh fruit and veggies and lots of long days with the sun beating down on your bare skin. Because we're all paying closer attention to the harmful effects of the sun, after another summer season, it's a great time to get to know your moles.

Moles are groupings of pigmented skin. An average adult usually has from ten to forty moles. A normal mole is one you've had since youth. It can be completely flat or dome shaped. A healthy mole is round and comes in one color.

Moles that you should get checked fall into the ABCD rule. A is for asymmetry. If you divided your mole in half, would one side look different from the other? B is for border. A mole that has a jagged or rough border is a bad sign. C is for color. This is for a mole with multiple colors or a change in color. D is for diameter. This means a mole bigger than one-quarter inch—roughly the size of the tip of an eraser. Most moles appear before you're thirty, so any new moles after that age warrant a little more attention. You should not be able to "feel" a mole—it should not itch or be sore unless you're irritating it with your clothing.

Many people are familiar with the moles they can see, but you need to know the moles on your back and everywhere else so you can be aware if they are changing. A mole may develop into malignant *melanoma*, "black mole cancer." When this mole gets to a certain thickness, it can spread to your insides. The key here is never getting to that point.

A good wide-brimmed sun hat would be a great investment on those sunny days. People who spend most of their time inside and get a "burst" of sun on days off are more likely to get sun cancer than those who live in the sun. So, weekend warriors especially need to cover up and slap on the sunscreen. If you're worried about putting chemicals on your skin, there are plenty of natural sunscreens out there. If your physician agrees that your mole looks a little scary, it can be removed. I promise you won't miss it.

This Might Scar

Just about everyone has at least one scar. For some, scars are a personal history book: "This one came from falling off a horse; that one on my knee came from an old football accident," and so on. Others can't stand scars. For them, scar tissue is painful, both physically and emotionally.

Why do we scar? We know that the body is smart, which means that scarring—which is ugly—must happen for a good reason. When our skin is broken, the scar is the last thing our body worries about. Its number-one priority is to guard against the threat of infection. As it rushes to repair itself, the body works against time. It doesn't waste its energy on neatness as it seals the open wound to keep out infection.

Other than ugly, is a scar tissue different from regular skin? Yes. On scar tissue, hair follicles and sweat glands do not grow back. Scarred skin is also less resistant to ultraviolet radiation, which means that you can burn more easily where your scar is. Scar tissue does not move or stretch the same way normal skin does; if a scar is over a joint, it can actually restrict movement.

A natural question would be that if skin renews itself, why does the scar stay? Scar tissue is knit together in a way that will not renew itself. If you got a scar when you were five, that scar tissue will stay with you the rest of your life.

Not all scars are the same. A typical scar is just a simple line. A widespread scar can occur after surgery or, in the case of stretch marks, when the skin becomes thinner and literally spreads out. There are two types of scars that occur when the body lays down too much tissue, and these are easy to spot because they are raised above the surrounding skin. They are called *hypertrophic* and *keloid* scars. The difference is that a keloid scar has no boundaries. It can grow to be much larger than the original injury. One can get a keloid scar the size of a quarter after something as small as a simple ear piercing. Scars can also appear in a sunken form, as from acne or chicken pox. And younger people are more likely to scar than older folks.

A scar is only a scar after the body's work is done, and there are some things you can do to minimize the look of the scar. First, never pick at scabbed tissue. This is nature's natural bandage. Second, cover up your scars with natural antimicrobial products like witch hazel or tea tree oil to reduce the visible effects. You can exfoliate once the skin is well on the healing path and increase your intake of vitamin C: both of these help reduce skin pigmentation problems.

Scars that Run Deep

Deep-tissue scarring, or *adhesions,* is a common complication from any significant assault to the body. An adhesion is a union of two or more tissues of the body. Infection, injury, surgery, or chemotherapy can cause the unnatural bonds that occur when wet tissue sticks together.

The body has plenty of wet tissue that glides past each other as you go about your daily activities. After an assault to the body, the natural response is inflammation, the defense mechanism that brings healing white blood cells to the front line. When this inflammation causes moist tissues to stick together and remain that way after the tissues have returned to their normal sizes, this becomes an adhesion that can be a tiny pinpoint or a thick, fibrous band.

Some adhesions don't bother us much, but others can be downright debilitating, depending on the location. An adhesion in your abdomen can cause a slowdown in digestion and create chronic pain. Adhesions are responsible for 60 percent of all bowel obstructions, for example. When the adhesion is in the pelvic region, infertility and ectopic pregnancies may result. An adhesion over the liver can make it difficult to breathe deeply. Free movement is essential to the body working right. Nerve endings may get tangled up within an adhesion, causing even further pain.

Some people have surgery to free up adhesions caused from earlier surgeries, but this doesn't always get rid of the problem: the body scars up again about 70 percent of the time. For this reason, most insurance companies won't cover these surgical procedures. Steps are being taken to minimize the risk of adhesions in surgery. Doctors are using the finest-sized sutures possible and doing their best to avoid introducing foreign materials—like the powder from surgical gloves—into the wound. Many massage therapists are trained in breaking up adhesions, but the work takes time. You won't solve the problem in one visit, but for those with chronic pain, this procedure is worth your time. An anti-inflammatory is usually recommended to help reduce the body's reaction. Be sure to ask your health-care provider about the natural choices available.

One of the most important aspects of healing is emotional and mental support. All too often, patients with chronic adhesion pain are told that, "It's all in your head." Knowledge is power. Awareness, understanding, and respect are crucial partners in wellness.

Toenail Fungus

When the warm weather comes, how happy we are to get out the summer shoes and expose our toes to the gentle breezes ... unless we are plagued by toenail fungus. Who wants to show off those thick, discolored nails to the world?

Those who have toenail fungus can actually lose the nail itself if the situation isn't treated. The challenge is that it can be tough to get rid of, so let's take a look at this phenomenon and find out how we come by it and what we can do to get rid of it.

Toenail fungus begins innocently enough as a white or yellow spot under the tip of your nail. It can spread deep into the nail and can infect neighboring nails. The fungus is at home in warm, moist environments like locker rooms, inside a stinky pair of sneakers, or around your favorite hot tub. You can get a fungal infection in your fingernails, too, but it's far less common because your hands aren't subject to the same environment as toes experience inside your shoes.

The fungus gets in through tiny cuts or through a small separation between your nail and nail bed. A nail with a fungal infection is thick, with crumbly edges, and can be yellow, green, brown, or black, depending on the color of the gunk that gets stuck behind it. In a really bad case, the nail can fall off and develop a foul odor.

A toenail infection can get quite painful and cause permanent damage to your nails. If you have diabetes, any minor problem in the foot can lead to a more serious complication. Since the fungus can spread from toe to toe, it's important to catch it early.

Over-the-counter treatments aren't very effective. Stronger, prescribed medications, while doing a better job of tackling a fungus, have side effects that range from skin rashes to liver damage. Homeopathic remedies include nutritional supplements and cold laser treatments, both of which we use in our office.

For those with pristine toes, here are some helpful hints to help keep them this way: don't go barefoot in public places; after exercising, take off your shoes and socks and let your feet breathe; remove nail polish to let the nail breathe; don't trim or pick at the skin around your nails—this is like putting out a welcome mat for fungus to get in.

Take action, and before you know it, you'll have toes that will make any sandal proud.

Warts: Yet Another Use for Duct Tape

"You're beautiful, warts and all."

Many of us have the noncancerous viral skin growths known as warts. We get them thanks to a virus called *HPV* that causes rapid growth of the outer layers of your skin. These painless residents usually make themselves at home on the hands of youngsters who are always touching everything. Although they usually go away on their own, most people don't want to wait. They come up with all sorts of weapons and strategies to send them packing—some of them are harmless and some are not so nice.

Warts are small, flesh-colored, grainy bumps that are much like scar tissue. They can occur in patches, or you can have just one. If you look closely, you may be able to see a few black tiny dots. These are commonly called "wart seeds," but are actually just clotted blood vessels.

Can you get a wart from touching a frog? Not likely. Common warts are spread from another person by touch. You can also spread the virus to other places on your body if you already have a wart. In either case, they need an invitation, which comes in the form of a break in your skin. The virus that causes warts can get in through openings like a hangnail, cut, or scrape.

To avoid spreading warts, don't use the same file or clipper on warts as you do on healthy nails. Clipping, combing, or shaving an area around a wart can also spread the virus. Picking at the wart can also give the virus wings, so hands off. It's also best to keep your hands as dry as possible as viruses spread best in moist environments.

But what about the duct tape? Salicylic acid patches used to be the standard way to go. Now the mainstream sources (including the Mayo clinic) recommend using duct tape, suggesting that it works even better than the medication.

Here is how to perform duct tape therapy:

Cover your wart with duct tape. After six days, remove the tape and soak the wart in water for a few minutes. Gently rub the wart with an emery board or pumice stone. Repeat this cycle for up to two months or until the wart is gone. The best theory as to why this works is that the tape irritates the skin and causes your immune system to go on the attack. The good news is that it's an inexpensive treatment that's a lot less scary to your children than *cryotherapy*, or freezing

Warts are generally harmless, and time heals all wounds, including warts.

Chapter Four:
Muscles

The human body is the only machine for which there are no spare parts.

~Hermann M. Biggs

Don't Let This Muscle Cramp Your Style

Your muscles hold down a highly skilled job. To get up out of a chair, entire groups of muscles have to relax while others have to contract in a symphony of motion whose timing must be exact. Your body masters this movement almost effortlessly, in spite of this fact.

Occasionally, your body's worker bees get out of sync, and unwanted muscle spasms, called muscle cramps, hit us. A muscle cramp, or *charley horse*, can last from just a few seconds to as long as fifteen minutes. The most common muscle to seize up is your *gastrocnemius*, located in the back of your lower leg. Next to go are the muscles in the back or front of your thighs, which are your *quads* or *hamstrings*. After that, any muscle under voluntary control is fair game. A cramp begins with a sharp and sudden pain that will stop you in your tracks. A rock-hard lump of muscle tissue can usually be seen just beneath the skin.

There are many causes of a muscle cramp: dehydration, overexertion, and injury are commonly the cause. One can also get a muscle cramp from not enough blood heading to the muscle or from a nerve being pinched. A loss of potassium (potassium levels fall from many blood pressure medications or any other diuretic) can also cause a muscle cramp.

If you get a muscle cramp, it's time for a time-out and a checklist. Are you getting enough water? A good way to tell is that your urine should be straw yellow, which has just a hint of yellow, almost clear. If you get leg cramps often, it might be from a nerve being pinched and in that case, getting adjusted should help. Another possibility is that you might not be stretching enough. If you get cramps during the night, start a stretching routine before bed. To help with circulation try a good massage.

Athletes are prone to get cramps in the preseason because their bodies aren't used to all the work. Whether you're a pro or not, it's best to gradually increase your workouts; don't just wake up one morning and decide to run five miles that day.

The body is a highly efficient machine whose needs are pretty simple. Sometimes a glass of water can be the most effective cure.

Tennis Anyone?

Tennis elbow is the more common term for *lateral epicondylitis*. If you stood with your palms facing forward, the outside half of your elbows would be the area we're talking about.

Tennis elbow is an inflammation of some of the tendons in your forearm. Tendons are like really strong ropes that anchor a muscle onto a bone. When these tendons become inflamed, the pain can begin outside the elbow and travel down to the wrist. You might notice a little bump where the pain starts, and you might have some trouble opening a pickle jar due to a weak grip.

"But I don't play tennis," you might say. That's okay. The condition is nicknamed tennis elbow because a poor backhand stroke can be one of many things that cause it. You can get it from many other repetitive activities, such as hammering, using a screwdriver, and painting, just to name a few. Any activity that uses the muscles that raise your hand and wrist is fair game.

If you have it and you're like most Americans, your preferred solution might be to ignore it and hope it goes away. Most of us try to work though the pain. Sometimes that works, but usually it just gets worse. For those who like to take action, the first step is a no-brainier. Since this is an overuse injury, the first thing to do is discontinue the activity that caused it. If the activity is something you do at work and you're not ready (or able) to take time off, some ergonomic steps might do the trick.

Ice the area. Elevate the elbow when you can, putting a pillow under the affected arm whenever possible and definitely when you're sleeping. If this doesn't make a difference, you might want to seek some outside help. A type of massage called *cross-fiber*, or friction, massage can speed up the healing process by increasing circulation if it has reached a chronic state. A chiropractor can look at the elbow to see if either of the bones in your forearm is out of place. If your elbow looks deformed, if you've had a major accident, or you have a fever, this is not tennis elbow and medical attention is in order.

If you got tennis elbow from playing tennis, you may wonder if your days on the court are over. After your elbow has calmed down, you can get back in the game. To stay out of trouble, however, try a lesson or two on improving your form.

Tenosynovitis … When Your Green Thumb
Turns Into a Painful Thumb

Tenosynovitis, also known as *De Quervan's tendonitis,* is an inflammation of the tendons at the base of your thumb. To explain it, let's take apart the word. "Teno" is short for tendons. Tendons are ropes that tie muscles to bones. In this case, these tendons are at the base of the thumb and make moving your thumb around possible. The "syno" part is short for *synovial sheath*. A sheath is a sleeve or pocket that lubricates all of these tendons and keeps everything moving freely. Finally, the "itis" part means there is an inflammation. When things are inflamed, they are larger than they should be. This limits the room the tendons have to move, and friction develops.

How can someone know they have this condition? The symptoms are pretty basic. Pain is felt at the base of the thumb; twisting the wrist is painful; using a screwdriver is out of the question. A good test for De Quervan's is *Finkelstein's test.* There are two parts to this test. First, you make a fist with your thumb on the inside (think of a "girl" fist). Then, you move your wrist down toward the pinky side of your hand in the same motion you'd use to cast a fishing lure. If this movement is pretty painful, we have a bingo here.

How would this condition develop? De Quervan's can be a side effect of pregnancy or it can develop in someone with rheumatoid arthritis, but most commonly it is caused by an overuse injury of the wrist. Typing, twisting—like with a screwdriver or trimming your hedges—can do this. Gardening can be particularly hard on the wrist and thumb.

If all this sounds familiar, you may want to know what can be done to help. In a simple procedure, the thumb is simply removed, with your good thumb left intact. Just kidding! Treatment is simple. First, since this is an overuse issue, cutting out what caused it is the first step. Sometimes people need to get a splint to get them to stop using their thumb and wrist. Since this is also an inflammation, putting ice on the swollen spot can speed healing. A good anti-inflammatory can help. (There are a lot of natural anti-inflammatory aids out there.) If this overuse injury came about because you've knocked your thumb out of place, a good gentle adjustment can put it back into proper alignment. If this is from pregnancy, you can do things to relieve the symptoms, but you won't be pregnant forever; after the baby comes the swelling will go down.

After all of this has calmed down and your painful swollen thumb has returned to its former self, you can put it back to work, but this time, be a little kinder to yourself.

Chapter Five:
Nerves

Sometimes your body is smarter than you are.

~Author Unknown

No Pain, no Gain?

You're walking along without a care in the world. It's a beautiful day. The sun is shining; the birds are chirping. Then you make a false step and stub your toe. Ouch! Your Birkenstocks do a lot of good in many ways, but unless you're wearing a new steel-toed variety, they don't offer much protection for your toes. Pain travels up from your toe and stops you in your tracks.

When your eyes clear and your hands unclench, you wonder how the brain knew what had happened so fast. You may also be wondering why the pain was so sharp and why some people feel pain differently than you do.

Let's go back to your poor, throbbing toe. The message relay system works on many levels, beginning with your skin. You have many receptors in your skin. Some tell your brain that your toe is cold or hot, some sense touch, others can tell that your shoe is too tight, and there are ones that let you know you're in pain. These receptors are concentrated in areas of the body that are prone to injury, like your fingers and toes. That's why a paper cut can be agony on your finger but not so bad someplace else.

So your toe gets crunched. Pain receptors send the message up the nerve they branch off from. This nerve joins the others in your back to form the spinal cord, sending the message to your brain. This whole process happens in the blink of an eye.

This process used to be the sum total of our knowledge about pain, but in time we realized that the human body is much more complicated than that. During World War II, doctors noticed that the degree of pain suffered by some wounded soldiers did not always correlate with how badly hurt they were. Researchers were inspired to dig deeper, and they discovered that there are sensory gatekeepers in your spine. The messages they decide are most important are allowed to get through, while others are left waiting at the gate.

Remember when your mom used to kiss your scraped knees, elbows, and shins when you were young? Her feel-good kiss blocked some of your pain thanks to the positive messages received by your body's sensory receptors. The brain received a mixed message that said, "I'm hurt, but help is at hand." You began to feel better very quickly after that.

Now let's look at the reasons the same pain stimulus can affect people differently. Your emotional state, your upbringing, and your attitude all come into play here, because a big part of the way we feel pain is connected to surprise, anger, and fear. As children, when we bumped our heads or fell, we shed tears of surprise. We hadn't expected to get hurt, and the shock was worse than the pain itself. Think of the person who has a poor track record with dentists. She will already be braced for the anticipated pain walking into the dentist office. On the flip side, people who have conditioned themselves to endure pain can easily handle experiences that would stop the rest of us dead in our tracks. Imagine trying to walk on hot coals the way firewalkers do—or sleeping on a bed of nails as a spiritual ritual without any of the proper conditioning! What the experts have done is program their sensory receptors to recognize pain and respond to it in ways that are different from ours. Like the healing kiss from your mom, their mental attitude sends a message to the brain saying, "I'm aware of this sensation; there's no need to panic."

Medical experts are learning more about pain all the time, which is good. It's an ongoing, uphill struggle to keep up with all the chronic conditions people suffer from. Knowledge is power. Now that you know how pain works, you also know that you can turn to your practitioner to help you identify your problems and work with you to deal with them.

Hiccup ... Hiccup ... Hiccup

There you were back in high school, taking the biggest test of your life. In an anything but cozy room you gripped your number 2 pencil. It was so quiet you could almost hear your brain sort through its mental files, looking for answers. Without warning, "Hiccup!" was released from your body. While you felt the glaring death rays from the students you disturbed, you were helpless to prevent the next one and the next and the next.

Hiccups never come at convenient times, and most of us can't explain what they are. All we know is that as soon as we get them, we want them gone.

To really understand the hiccup, we need to talk nerves. I like to think of the nervous system as the electric wiring of the body. Just as in your home, your nerves branch off to deliver power to different places. All of these nerves are named, even the one responsible for hiccups. The *vagus* nerve runs from your brain down to your belly, with many stops in between. The vagus nerve is not the shy, quiet type. If any of the part of the digestive system that it controls becomes irritated, it will tweak a nearby *phrenic* nerve. The phrenic goes to the dome-shaped muscle under your lungs called the *diaphragm*. The tweak causes the diaphragm to go into spasm, causing the "hiccup" sound.

There's got to be at least a hundred cures for hiccups, but they generally fall into one of two camps: cures that overstimulate the vagus nerve and cures that interfere with breathing.

To confuse the vagus nerve, place a spoonful of sugar at the back of your tongue, where sour sensation normally takes place. Another good vagus distraction is to gargle with saltwater.

The other type of cure gives the body something bigger to focus on by decreasing oxygen and upping carbon dioxide levels. Everything from breathing into a brown paper bag to just plain holding your breath fits into this category. I'm a pretty big fan of breathing deeply, so my personal preference is the spoonful of sugar.

With the body, even the simplest responses pack a pretty complex explanation. And we've just scratched the surface as to what makes us tick.

Sciatica

If you suddenly start feeling pain in your lower back or hip that radiates downward from your buttock to the back of one thigh and into your leg, your problem may be *sciatica*, an irritation of the sciatic nerve.

The most common cause of sciatica is a slipped or protruding disc that is putting pressure on the sciatic nerve. Discs are the cushions that act as shock absorbers and separate the bones of the spine. Discs can be compared to a jelly- or cream-filled donut: the outside is tough and fibrous, while the center is soft and pliable. If part of the outer surface is weak, the center may push through. We feel pain when a protruding disc presses on our sciatic nerve, the longest nerve in the body. The pain is usually worse if you sit, sneeze, or cough. It can feel like a weakness, numbness, burning, or tingling sensation that sometimes goes all the way to your toes.

The nerves transmit messages around the body. We can tell whether something is hot or cold from the messages our nerves send to our brain. Conversely, our brain can use the nerves to send messages to the muscles, causing them to contract.

Most of the time, sciatica is not a serious condition. Though the pain may be extreme, the situation usually sorts itself out within a few weeks. There are many natural treatment options available, and only a very small percentage of cases require surgery. That being said, if you experience progressive weakness or incontinence with sciatica, you should seek medical attention immediately.

The pain from sciatica may be severe enough to keep you in bed for a few days. When it begins to subside, you should try to be as active as possible to help minimize the pain: inactivity actually makes the pain worse.

Your low back muscles and core muscles need to be stretched and strengthened to enable them to support your back. Ask your health-care practitioner for specific exercises for the low back and abdomen. Exercise will help keep nutrients and fluids moving in and out of those discs too.

You should also go to your chiropractor to confirm that your condition truly is sciatica and have her perform adjustments needed to realign bones and relieve pressure on the sciatic nerve.

Small, everyday, preventative measures include not standing in one place for extended periods; not sitting with your wallet in your back pocket; and not wearing high heels. If you have to stand on the job, get a footrest and alternate propping up one foot, then the other. Take your wallet out of your back pocket when you're going to be sitting for extended periods. Don't wear high heels for long periods, if you must wear them at all.

Sciatica can be very painful, but it can be successfully treated if you take notice of it before too much damage is done. Think of it as a wake-up call, a chance to start listening to your body and take care of it.

Carpal Tunnel Syndrome

Almost everyone knows someone who's dealt with wrist and hand problems, often diagnosed as carpal tunnel syndrome. Your hands fall asleep or become painful, you lose grip strength, you can't hold a pen long enough to write a letter or, worse yet, type one. In this article, we're going to take a closer look at carpal tunnel and what to do about it.

First let's back up and talk about nerves. Nerves carry impulses from the brain to the nerve endings and from the nerve endings to the brain. Nerves usually get into trouble at the joints where they are most exposed and vulnerable. When you hit your funny bone at the elbow, you're actually hitting your *unlar* nerve and getting a shock down the arm.

In the case of carpal tunnel, it is the *median* nerve getting pinched at the wrist. The median nerve can also get in trouble as it crosses the elbow, shoulder, and the base of the neck where it joins the spinal cord. This means that someone can have a problem in the neck that is causing trouble in the hand or a problem in the wrist that is causing trouble in the neck, or both. This is called *double crush* syndrome.

So how does a nerve get pinched at a joint? In the case of carpal tunnel, the nerves and vessels are squeezed at the wrist as they pass through a tunnel formed by bones and tendons. Nerve entrapment may develop from trauma to the wrist, such as forcefully bending the wrist backward, or just from daily work habits like hammering, typing, or any repetitive motion where the wrist is bent backward. The earlier you can diagnose and treat the problem, the easier it is to fix and avoid surgery. Sometimes a wrist brace is necessary as well as nutritional supplements, especially a balanced supply of B6.

Chiropractic helps with carpal tunnel by fixing the tunnel and freeing the nerve. Imagine crimping a garden hose and finding that only a trickle of water is coming out, even though the spigot is wide open. This is what happens to the hands with carpal tunnel. By adjusting the bones in the wrist and arm, the "hose" gets uncrimped.

This analogy also explains how chiropractic works in general. As chiropractors, we believe that there is a universal force that flows through us and breathes life into us. We all know how good it feels when we're in the flow, and we also know how it feels when we're blocked. These blocks manifest in us physically, emotionally, mentally, and energetically. In chiropractic we call this a subluxation, which means literally, a state of less than perfect light. The goal of chiropractic adjustment is to remove blocks in the body, allowing the light to shine.

Chapter Six:
Joints

Diagnosis is not the end, but the beginning of practice.

~Martin H. Fischer

That Bump Is a Bunion

The joint that connects your big toe to your foot can become a very tender place. It can become red and swollen and harden over time. It can make walking a pain and kill any dreams of ever becoming a sandal model. Today, bunions are way too common (over half of American women have them), so let's figure out how that painful bump got there in the first place and what we can do to straighten things out.

The word "bunion" comes from the French word for "turnip." Bunions can develop a reddened painful sack over them that, in the right light, can look like a turnip. With a bunion comes a bulging bump on the inside of the big toe. This bump isn't extra fluid or swollen tissue: it's the base of your big toe changing direction. Instead of pointing straight ahead, your big toe leans in toward the second toe, causing crowding. This crowding can turn into a pretty painful situation and make you not want to leave the couch. Over time, you can lose range of motion in your toe.

How did this bunion come to be? There are two likely culprits. First, there is your foot itself. When normal balance is interrupted, abnormal stress is placed on the joint in your foot. Take being flatfooted for example. When you have a nice arch, part of your foot hits the ground first just like a graceful swan dive. When you're flatfooted, your whole foot hits the ground all at once, like a big belly flop. All that extra pressure has to go somewhere.

The second probable cause is what you put on your foot. Shoes that squeeze the toes together can bring about a bunion. High heels and shoes that are just plain too tight can become big problems.

The good news is that a bunion does not happen overnight, so prevention should be easy. When shoe shopping, look for shoes with at least a half- inch space between the tip of your longest toe and the end of your shoe, and avoid shoes that come to a point. It's also good to get your foot adjusted if you suspect something has gone out of place.

If you already have a bunion, there are steps you can take to help yourself. Any time your bunion is red and swollen apply, ice to help calm it. Wearing a pad on the bunion can protect it from further irritation. Over-the-counter arch supports are also worth a shot. If the pain persists, a visit to your trusted health-care professional can give you more options for relief and healing.

Before you wedge your foot into those pretty high heels, just remember that the "price of fashion" may be higher than you bargained for.

Your discs and Jelly Donuts

Did we mention donuts just to get your attention? Actually, jelly is a perfect example when comparing something familiar to the discs in your spine. Even better, jelly helps explain what is happening when your discs come under pressure and start to bulge outward.

The spine is an elegant compromise in form and function. To achieve the range of motion your neck and back require, a little bit of stability has been sacrificed. Your spine has twenty-four bones stacked on top of one another. In between those bones, acting like cushiony pillows, are the discs that keep the bones from grinding against each other when you turn you head, swing your golf club, or bend your waist. The ligaments are the ropes that lock these bones together, while the muscles use tendons to grab hold of the bones. The muscles are the movers and shakers at the party. And last but not least, we have the nerves, which use the spine as their freeway to get messages to and from the brain.

Okay, back to the jelly donut. Like our calorie-laden friend, discs have two layers. The jelly, or nucleus, sits safely in the center. Just as the donut crust keeps the jelly from getting all over your hands, your *annulus* is the tough outer layer that holds everything in place.

When a disc is herniated, the donut crust becomes weak, and the soft center spills out. A bulging disc is what we get when a weak spot bulges out due to internal pressure. What causes it to bulge is sometimes hard to pin down. In some cases, it can be traced back to a specific incident: lifting something heavy or maybe a car accident. Most of the time, it's just a case of wear and tear; our discs age just like the rest of our body, getting tired and worn after years of working overtime.

The usual suspects for _disc degeneration_ are in the neck and lower back. How this is felt depends on the location. In your lower back, the disk can set the _sciatic nerve_ on fire, shooting a pain right down the back of your leg. A disc problem at the base of the neck may be felt all the way down to your fingertips.

Why you feel numbness, tingling, and more is because discs are the spacers of the back, keeping a healthy distance between your backbones. When they degenerate, they shrink and the bones get too close for comfort. The nerves that use these spaces as tunnels to send signals feel the squeeze and let you know that trouble is at hand.

Some people end up going under the knife, but most of the time this can be avoided. Simple disc bulges can be managed with chiropractic care. For many, decompression therapy is their best option. Computer-controlled tension can distract a disc back into place, suction nutrients and oxygen back into the disc and retract the bulging or hernia, returning the disc to its healthy roots.

Some people will try to ignore the problem until the pain becomes too severe and they find themselves held hostage to it. If you're staying in on a perfectly good golf day or your choice of shoes are the ones you don't have to bend over to put on, you aren't managing the pain: it's keeping you from living.

Get on the Good Foot

Your feet endure a tremendous amount of shock throughout the day. Their makeup includes several irregularly shaped bones held together by a web of muscles, tendons, ligaments, and thick fascia. They usually work together in a complex, harmonious fashion, but when they fail, they can cause tremendous pain with every step: pain that can spread up to the knees and low back.

One of the most common foot problems is that of *pronation*, more commonly known as being flatfooted. Foot pronation is when some of the bones in the foot roll inward, causing the foot to lose its structural integrity. Normally, the tendon in the back of your ankle (your Achilles) should line up with the calf. With foot pronation, the Achilles migrates from the center toward the other foot. When looking head-on at someone with foot pronation, it may look like they are walking on the insides of their feet. If you have had pain in your feet and ankles for a while, you can check for pronation by looking at an old pair of shoes. The soles of your shoes should be worn down evenly. With foot pronation, the insides of the soles wear down first, and your shoes tend to collapse inward. Another way to check is when standing: see if there is any weight placed on the inside arch of your feet.

Foot pronation does not only affect the feet and ankles. When the ankle is out of line, the knee rotates toward the midline, making your kneecaps point toward each other rather than straight ahead. This will affect the way you walk, sending stress to your lower back.

One way to protect your feet is to make sure that the shoes you house them in are a good fit for your feet. Remember, not all feet are created equally, so a shoe that is supportive for your neighbor might not be right for you. Try this simple muscle test the next time you try on a pair of shoes. First, while you're barefoot, lace your fingers together and hold your arms out parallel to the ground with your elbows straight, like you would in volleyball. Have a friend press down on your forearms and see how long you're able to keep your arms up. Next, try the same experiment with the shoes on and see if you're as strong as you were barefoot. If you're any weaker, these aren't the shoes for you. The weakness shows how much energy and strength these shoes are actually taking from you.

You can also visit your chiropractor and make sure the bones in your foot are properly lined up. Rolling your ankle, stepping on a kids' Hot Wheel car, and poor shoes are just a few of the ways to knock a bone out of place. Once you get them back in place, you need to exercise and stretch the muscles in your feet and ankles so you can stay balanced and strong.

Shoulder Trouble

What most people refer to as the "shoulder" is really several joints working with tendons, muscles, and ligaments to allow a wide range of motion for the arms. The shoulder has amazing mobility that we often abuse, and soft tissue is injured. Soft-tissue injury sends a painful message that tells us something is wrong.

Imagine how many times you move your arms every day. Consider that every time you move your arms, your shoulder joints move too. It's not very surprising, when you stop and think about it, that shoulder problems can develop simply as a result of everyday wear and tear as well as from specific injuries.

The shoulder is a ball-and-socket joint, very much like the hip joint. While the hip is one of the most stable joints in the body, the shoulder is more fragile—rather like a golf ball perched on a tee. The clavicle is the tee, providing a very shallow socket for the ball of the arm bone to rest in.

The other half of the equation in shoulder movement is the soft tissue. This includes muscles, tendons, and ligaments that hold the bones together. Tendons are tough, ropelike fibers that connect muscle to bone; ligaments are fibers that connect bone to bone and help stabilize the joints. These fibers have to be tough enough to keep everything in place, yet pliable enough to maintain full range of motion.

There are over twenty muscles directly or indirectly involved in all the actions of the shoulder, making very complex integration necessary. When lifting a cup, for example, the muscles in the front of your arm must contract. At the same time, the muscles in the back of your arm must relax. The muscles, tendons, ligaments, bones, and nerves must work together in a complex symphony to maintain proper movement. Any imbalance will wreak havoc.

The shoulder has the greatest range of motion of any joint in the body. Because of this mobility, the shoulder is at a high risk for injury. One rule I like to go by is this: if you are wondering, "Can I lift this by myself?" you probably should get some help.

Avoid catching a falling object: the jarring motion of stopping the object can put unwanted tension on your joints. If your hand is outstretched far enough that it is beyond your peripheral vision, your shoulder is in a compromising position. A common example of this is when we reach for something in the backseat of the car while the seat belt holds our body in place.

If you hurt your shoulder, first aid is essential. The acronym RICE outlines the steps you need to follow: rest the injured area, ice the area to decrease swelling and internal bleeding, compress the area with an elastic bandage, elevate the injured part above the level of the heart to promote drainage of fluids from the area.

Until the fountain of youth is discovered, the best practice is to stay hydrated by drinking plenty of water and take glucosamine to promote ease of movement in the joints.

Fluid-filled sacs located around the joints lubricate the area to promote ease of movement. These sacs are called *bursa*. When they become irritated and swollen, the condition is called bursitis. The most commonly affected area is the shoulder, although you can also experience it in your elbow, hip, or knee. When the joint is out of alignment, bursitis can develop. Getting it adjusted will reduce the irritation, ease the inflammation, and return the joint to normal function.

The bicep is the muscle located in the front of your arm. It is connected to the bone by a tendon that sits in a groove. A sudden jar while the bicep muscle is contracted can cause a slipped *bicipital tendon*. When the tendon slips out of the groove, the tendon can become irritated. An example of this is when you are working together with someone to carry a heavy load, and the other person suddenly drops his end. The pain is felt in the upper front area of the arm.

Sometimes the muscles attempting to lift the arm are incapable of doing so because the muscles acting in opposition fail to relax at the appropriate time. This is one of the main causes of frozen shoulder syndrome: a loss of mobility that prevents the person from raising their arm above a certain point. It can be caused by ligament inflammation, arthritis, or bursitis. The secret to getting mobility back is finding and treating the underlying cause.

You can also injure or tear a ligament, dislocate the clavicle, or have arthritis in your shoulder. You may have an irritated nerve at the base of your neck or be experiencing referred pain from an internal organ.

Whatever is ailing you, it's important that you have your shoulder checked out and become an active partner in the healing process. Proper chiropractic care is an important part of a preventive maintenance program, too.

Got TMJ Disorder? Pass the Applesauce!

What's your favorite food? Is it a crisp apple right off the tree? How about a big burger that you have to open your mouth really wide to fit in? Maybe it's something sweet and chewy, like caramel candies.

For some people, these foods are painful to think about. It's not that they don't taste good; it's that it hurts too much to eat them. When it hurts enough that you can't chew anything, your next meal might look more like baby food. TMJ disorder (that's *temporomandibular joint disorder*) is a technical way of saying pain in your jaw joint.

Your jaw is called your mandible, and the bone it connects to in your skull is your temporal bone. These joints sit right in front of the ear. In between these bones sit discs like the ones between your backbones, but on a much smaller scale. These tiny discs skate around the joint, keeping the bones from banging together and the pressure evenly distributed. The jaw is considered a hinge joint, like the knee. Unlike the knee, your jaw moves from side to side and back to front for chewing, swallowing, and talking.

With so many complicated movements asked of the joint, much can go wrong. Both joints need to be working together for smooth movement. In some cases, the disc can slide out of place; you'll know this has happened when you can hear a clicking sound. The jaw itself can be out of place; this can be caused by many things, including, grinding our teeth at night, dental work, excessive gum chewing, and the occasional sucker punch.

A TMJ sufferer's jaw is usually tender, with an aching around the ear. Sometimes you can hear a clicking or grating sound when the mouth is opening. Someone with TMJ cannot "open wide," and when the situation gets really bad, the mouth may be stuck open or closed. Tough foods are off the menu because chewing hard foods can be excruciating.

Fixing this problem can involve a little detective work. If it began after a dental procedure, you may want to go back and make sure your bite is even. If the jaw or discs are out of place, a chiropractor can put them back in, just as they can with any bone. For those who grind their teeth in their sleep—your partner will tell you this sounds like fingernails on a chalkboard—doing something relaxing before bed can release the day's stress. Many massage therapists can work out those tight little muscles in there.

TMJ can be painful, but if you put yourself first and get help, you'll be eating an apple a day in no time.

This Kind of Joint You Don't Want

We have all heard the term *arthritis* thrown around, but do we really know what it is? It is often used as a catch-all term that seems to cover a broad range of symptoms, but it may not be appropriate to describe what is actually wrong. I say this because the term "arthritis" is generally misused and misunderstood by the public. Even doctors sometimes use the term too loosely.

Arthritis comes from the Greek "arthron," meaning joint, and "itis," meaning inflammation; thus, "arthritis" simply means the inflammation of a joint. The inflammation can range from mild, like a bug bite, to a very severe disease. You can create inflammation simply by scratching an itch or rubbing your skin. If the irritation is severe enough to cause redness along with some fluid accumulation, heat, and pain, you have inflammation.

The true meaning of the word "arthritis" describes a strain in a joint that then becomes swollen. This certainly doesn't mean that it's incurable; in fact, if left alone, the body will often cure itself. So why does the general public see arthritis as an incurable condition that has to be controlled with pain medication or smelly creams?

Because there are many types of arthritis, it is less than wise to take drugs to override the joint pain, allowing the condition to remain and possibly get worse. While we think of pain as the enemy, in reality it is our alarm system telling us when something is wrong. If there is smoke in your house and your smoke alarm is going off, do you take out the batteries to get rid of the annoying sound and go back to what you were doing? I hardly think so. Yet, we routinely reach for pain meds to dull our alarm signals when they go off so that we can go on with our day and ignore what's really going on.

There are records of people who have totally lost the ability to feel any pain thanks to prolonged use of pain inhibitors. This may sound like a pretty good deal, but with a little deeper inspection, you'll realize that it is actually devastating. Not only can these people hurt themselves without knowing it, they actually wear their weight-bearing joints down to bone-on-bone, because the body has no way to tell whether its joints are functioning properly.

As chiropractors, we often see patients who say they have arthritis, yet a thorough evaluation that includes muscle testing reveals no damage or disease process in the joint. The joint is simply in strain during movement, and when the joint's movement is returned to normal with a gentle adjustment, the pain is often immediately removed.

This type of joint strain is generally caused by improper muscle balance. If the muscles holding a joint are very weak on one side compared to the muscles on the other side, the joint is under constant strain. The person is thus in constant pain.

Osteoarthritis: Good Old Wear and Tear

Many types of arthritis respond favorably to treatment, while some can only be managed effectively if the condition is treated before severe damage develops. It's important to understand that if you've been diagnosed with arthritis, it may not be necessary to endure it. Certain types may be incurable, but certainly not all forms. When a doctor diagnoses arthritis, the patient often thinks the worst, resorting to pain pill override. This may be an unfortunate mistake.

The most common type of arthritis around is called *osteoarthritis* (OA), or degenerative joint disease. It's generally considered the "wear and tear" type of arthritis. It usually occurs from your fifties on and is most commonly found in the weight-bearing joints like the knees and hips. Another common location is in the hands, especially for people like carpenters, mechanics, and gardeners, among others. OA can develop as a result of injury. It is not the type of arthritis that migrates around the body from joint to joint.

Because OA is caused by joint strain, common sense dictates that you should find ways to remove strain from the joint to remove the problem. One obvious way is to keep your weight down. Another is to keep your joints in proper alignment so their mechanical functioning works correctly. Imagine wearing a fifty-pound backpack and then walking along the side of a hill for twenty miles. Do you think maybe your back or knees might hurt after a while? This example isn't very different from being overweight and walking in bad shoes for a few years.

Specific metabolic and nutritional deficiencies also contribute to OA by causing a weakening of the joint surfaces and making them vulnerable to wear and tear. Protein deficiency has been linked with having OA, too. This doesn't necessarily mean that you need to kick the tofu for a big steak; it's more likely that the body is failing to absorb the protein it's getting. Clues that protein may not be getting digested can include episodes of gas after a meal, brittle and cracking fingernails, and poor quality hair, to name a few.

Long-term OA usually shows calcium buildup in the joints, often forming bone spurs that grow into the joint (ouch!). Oftentimes, nutritional or supplemental additions of magnesium, potassium, and other minerals are necessary because the body absorbs calcium in different ways.

OA can become so severe that the pain becomes intolerable and surgery is the only resort. Surgical replacement with an artificial joint is becoming more common in the hip and other joints, and though it's a remarkable feat of surgery, it's obviously better to prevent it from going that far, if at all possible.

An interesting correlation has been made in the treatment of OA with chiropractic and muscle testing. Oftentimes, an individual who has X-ray evidence of a badly damaged joint as a result of OA will come in for treatment. In an effort to stop the condition's progress, the patient's joint structure will be balanced with muscle-balancing techniques and manipulation.

Many times the pain can be completely relieved, although the joint structure still appears damaged on an X-ray. The point is, although the damage to joint structure is permanent, the pain can still be relieved, so don't throw in the towel! By reducing weight and structural strain and improving nutritional and metabolic processes, the further advancement of OA can be markedly reduced or halted.

Rheumatoid Arthritis: A Civil War

We don't really know why people get *rheumatoid arthritis* (RA). It is an autoimmune disease in which the body attacks its own *synovial* tissue, preventing it from secreting lubricating fluid for the joints and bursa in the body.

If we think of a joint as the working ends of two toilet plungers sealed together, with the handles being the bones and the space between the plungers being the joint cavity, synovial tissue lines this joint cavity and keeps it filled with fluid to cushion and lubricate the joint. RA attacks this tissue, causing the joint to become inflamed, painful, stiff, and eventually, deformed.

RA begins to affect people earlier in life than osteoarthritis, occurring typically between forty and fifty years of age, and it's three times more prevalent in women. The first appearance of RA is usually after a severe infection or some form of stress. RA attacks the hands and feet first and then moves to the trunk, migrating from joint to joint as it progresses, often leaving deformities in its wake. The most prominent complaints are joint pain, tenderness, swelling, and stiffness, especially in the morning. This stiffness is called a "jelling" phenomenon.

The course and prognosis of the disease is unpredictable, and the average patient can expect periods of remission and flare-ups with a gradual worsening of disability and deformity. Poor adrenal gland function appears to have some causation in RA's development. The adrenal cortex manufactures anti-inflammatory and pro-inflammatory hormones that help control the inflammatory processes in the body. For this reason, artificial steroids used to be a common treatment to control RA, but replacing a natural function of the body has its drawbacks.

When the body receives adrenalin or any hormone externally, the organs responsible for making that hormone become weaker; eventually the person becomes totally dependent on the drug. Ideally, it's better to obtain proper adrenal gland function by boosting the adrenal glands naturally, providing the right balance of anti-inflammatory hormones. If the adrenal glands are exhausted and incapable of handling their functions, it is important to eliminate or minimize the stresses—physical, chemical, emotional, and thermal—with which the adrenal glands must work.

Chiropractors test the adrenal gland functions using muscle testing as part of a regular visit and supply nutritional support when needed. Adequate protein intake and digestion are essential, as is a balanced rationing of calcium with other body minerals. These factors help keep the bones and joints healthy to better resist inflammatory attacks. Keeping the nervous system running clear and all of our joints in proper alignment is an important step to obtaining optimal health.

Gouty Arthritis

When most people think of gout, they envision a fat guy with a swollen, painful big toe. This is a pretty good visual in one respect: roughly 95 percent of gout sufferers are male, overweight, and middle-aged. Although gout is extremely painful in the feet and big toe, it may occur in most any joint, tendon, finger, and even the kidney. It tends to roam before settling in a specific joint.

The common cause of gout is tiny, needle-like crystals of uric acid accumulating in the blood and body fluids. These crystals are like crushed glass that cut into bone and tissue and cause the rapid onset of excruciating tenderness, redness, swelling, and sometimes chills and fever. The crystals are most often caused by overeating, especially too much red meat, refined food, alcohol, sugar, or caffeine. So, folks following the Atkins/South Beach high protein diets need to be careful. Even if you're thin, poor metabolism can allow accumulations of uric acid that the overloaded kidney can't excrete properly into the urine.

Gout is considered a chronic lifetime disease once it is present. If not kept under control, gradual joint destruction will occur with longer and longer attacks. Diet is obviously very important with gouty arthritis, meaning that avoiding high-protein foods and heavy alcohol intake are critical. In some cases, the bowel is involved, and its action, along with normal bacterial count, must be improved. For this reason, some other changes may include nutritional supplements.

The bottom line in all arthritic conditions is to determine exactly what is taking place and eliminate the causative factors. This makes much more sense than overriding the discomfort with pain medication. Many people with arthritis correct the condition and lead happy, healthy lives.

Chapter Seven:
Bones

Parents are the bones on which children cut their teeth.

~Peter Ustinov

Bone Spurs: The Thorn in Your Spine

Our bones go through many changes. We're born into this world with small, soft, cartilage-filled bones. In no time (ask any mom), our bones are full size and rock hard. Some of us might think that our bones go into retirement by the time we reach adulthood. This is not true. Our bones are active construction sites, renewing bone tissue all the time.

Just because they can't build up anymore does not mean they don't build out. When bones do build out it's called a bone spur. This sharp, thorn-like projection can be formed on any bone and become quite painful—though the pain may not be evident at first. Some may not cause any trouble at all—you may not realize you have them until you see them on an X-ray. Others can be a nightmare. How they bother you will depend on where they take up residence in your body.

Let's say they are in your neck. You might have trouble breathing or swallowing. They can also push on a vein, restricting blood flow to the brain. If the spur is in your spine, you might feel numbness down the course of a nerve and get a "pins and needles" sensation running down to your toes. In your fingers, you may be able to "see" the spurs from the outside as hard lumps under the skin. Wherever there's a bone in the body, a spur can form, and they can damage whatever they can find to needle.

Why does the body do this? In some cases, a bone spur can actually be beneficial. Normally, bones are connected by a joint with cushy cartilage at both ends of the bones. Over the years, this cartilage can begin to wear down, bringing the two bones in the joint too close for comfort. In a case like this, the bones do what they can to band-aid the situation, forming new bone around the edges of the existing bone. These spurs actually help areas of cartilage that are breaking down or help redistribute the weight.

The best way to avoid spur issues is not to give the body a reason to build a spur in the first place. Translation: protect your joints. Drink plenty of water. Many of us are slightly shorter at the end of each day: this is because our joints shrivel up due to dehydration. If your bones are out of alignment, joints age faster due to uneven wear and tear. The supplement glucosamine can give your body the ingredients necessary to begin rebuilding the cartilage. You may also want to look into some natural products to reduce inflammation.

You may not always like it or agree with it, but your body always has a reason for what it does. Why not be good to it and give it a reason to do better?

The Hip Bone Is Connected to the Knee Bone

What a fun childhood song. What a good way to get the little ones moving. They also learn the names of body parts while they're busy having fun.

What about us? Is there anything we can learn from this song? What about the message that the body is connected and that one part affects the other? That when you walk around on a bad knee favoring one leg, your hips will eventually be affected? The parts of the body that are close together are more than just neighbors: they must work together, too.

Maybe you have a "bum" knee. Could be from an old football injury or it's just overworked from all of your exciting adventures. Eventually, the hip will get dragged into the picture if you don't take care of things, if you're way too busy and too independent to seek care.

The bad knee will pull other bones out of place, causing uneven wear and tear on the joint. Muscles in your leg will be pulling as they try to stabilize the area. Your good knee has to bear more weight than it signed up for. Next thing you know, you're moving your hips differently. The rhythm you perfected since you crawled out of diapers and into short pants is out of sync. Now the hip begins to hurt, and instead of a "bad" knee, you now have a "bad" leg.

Suppose the knee is not the cause of the problem but the victim. Many people are flatfooted. What this means to your knee is that a flat foot does not land softly, supported by an arch. It smacks the ground, sending shock waves up the legs to knees and beyond. Being flatfooted also means that you tend to stand on the "insides" of your feet, pulling your knees out of line and closer together. To stop the problem before it takes over completely, get your knee put back in place, massaged, and worked on. Take your glucosamine to rebuild the joint.

Let's Bone Up on Osteoporosis

In most cases, it's pretty insulting to be called "dense," but when the subject of your bones is on the table, you can take dense as a complement. How our skeletons tip the scale might not seem to be too high on your priority list, especially since our bones tend to stay out of sight and out of mind. But without good strong bones to keep all our parts organized, we would soon fall flat on our faces. The term that describes bones that are beginning to fail is *osteoporosis*.

To understand osteoporosis, we need to know how a bone is designed. A bone is not completely solid, through and through. It has a hard outer shell that surrounds a honeycomb on the inside. "Osteo" means bone, and "porosis" is translated into porous. If we could peak inside bones that have osteoporosis, we'd see the honeycomb matrix wasting away and the spaces between growing larger. These tiny holes in your bones eventually expand until they connect to each other, creating tunnels that undermine the strength of your bones. When the hard outer core begins to disintegrate, you're left with hardly a leg to stand on.

Anyone can get osteoporosis, but women are most vulnerable. Women of short stature (less bone to start with), light-skinned people, those with a poor diet, and couch potatoes top the list.

Calcium is a key ingredient in our bones and a major player in blood chemistry. Think of the calcium in our blood as a checking account, while the calcium in our bones represents our savings. If you're not getting enough calcium in your diet, your blood will draw what it needs from the calcium saved in your bones. Too many withdrawals, and the savings account will be drained and your bones will look like Swiss cheese.

The seeds of osteoporosis can be traced back to our twenties and thirties, when we reach our peak bone mass. This is the most calcium we'll ever have on deposit, and as time passes, the body gradually depletes the supply. Fortunately, we have the ability to slow this depletion.

When it comes to your bones, the phrase "Use it or lose it" rings true. Exercise and an active lifestyle give your bones a reason to build thick walls. This means that by increasing your daily activity, you can begin to rebuild. Eat plenty of calcium as part of a healthy diet. Potassium, magnesium, vitamin D, and sunshine are all essential ingredients, too. Eat a balanced diet, which includes all these nutrients, and think of vitamins as your health insurance plan.

We all hope to live long lives. Let's keep our bodies healthy so the years can be full ones, too.

Break a Leg ... Stress Fractures

Hips are broken every day from bad falls. Ribs are often broken in car accidents. Sports like motocross cause your bones to shudder. Bones can break in one spot or shatter into many pieces. In a young person, they can bend in what is called a *greenstick fracture*. With *stress fractures*, no big-bang accident causes them, and for that reason, they can often be overlooked.

There are two ways to get a stress fracture: it takes an abnormal bone or an abnormal stress to manifest.

Osteoporosis (when your bones become porous like Swiss cheese) is a good example of abnormal bone. When the bone is weak or malnourished, everyday activity is stressful to the body. Something simple like a light fall can cause a stress fracture in this case.

The other way to get a stress fracture is reserved for those weekend-warrior types. Runners and long-distance hikers are top candidates here. Repetitive action plus muscle fatigue are a bad combination. Normally when you're walking, your muscles absorb most of the shock, but they eventually they get tired. When we don't rest our muscles at this point, the bones are left to fend for themselves. Try as they might, bones are not good shock absorbers, and eventually a stress fracture forms.

How could you have a fracture and not even know it? A stress fracture is not a clean break. Picture a bunch of tiny cracks together on a spot on a bone. Just like a house with a crumbling foundation, you don't see it from the outside. It takes an X-ray to confirm that it's there.

How can you tell otherwise? You'd probably feel pain that is worse after a workout. The skin around the fracture would be swollen and hurt to the touch. Unfortunately, these symptoms can be easily mistaken for something else, like shin splints.

Once you get a stress fracture, what do you do about it? Most important: do nothing. Get plenty of rest and follow you doctor's advice. (This may sound easy, but active people who get stress fractures hate sitting around.) Crutches, ice, and splints are often part of the picture, too. If you have to stay off your feet for long, some physical therapy would be beneficial to rebuild your stability. You might need an adjustment after limping around. After you've healed, remember to warm up and stretch to keep it from happening again.

Like many things in nature, the body likes variety. Cross train and vary your workout. Life is all about finding a balance between your ambition and how far your body is ready to go.

About the Authors

The doctor of the future will give no medicine but will interest his patients in the care of the human frame, in diet and in the cause and prevention of disease.

~ Thomas Edison

When Christine and I first arrived in our new hometown and opened our chiropractic clinic, we were following in the footsteps of a local legend. He had become both a trusted professional and a valued friend to the people he served over the years, and we saw the value that this relationship added to his life, and theirs.

Relationships are all about giving. We felt that we could give something of value to our community by writing articles that would be educational and informative—short summaries that would provide the reader with a better understanding of the active role they can play in improving their health.

Knowledge is power. The more someone knows, the more empowered they become. We've met patients with diabetes who could find their medicine in their purse blindfolded but have no idea what foods might make those pills unnecessary. We realized that people know how to live sick. We want them to learn how to live well.

There is no reason people shouldn't be able to understand important health issues, and through the articles we've written, we invite them to absorb the information at their own pace, in their own time. We try to communicate in a way that people can understand and enjoy, rather than feel threatened or challenged. Our articles have a light tone and simple language that make learning fun. During office visits, time is short. This is a big reason why so many health-care professionals have difficulty communicating, much less teaching their patients. By writing our weekly articles, we reach a large market and relay our information in a format that is a pleasure to read.

Our market has grown over the years. Most people tell us that they're curious about health topics and want to be knowledgeable but couldn't get past the "medical jargon" or get a clear, understandable answer from their doctor. They tell us that our articles made them feel smarter, because they could understand what we were telling them. They tell us that they look forward to each new column, because they've come to think of us as their personal advisers and friends.

We are honored and grateful for their continued support and hope that you will have fun reading this collected edition. We hope you will come away feeling empowered, because you have gained a better understanding about your health and how it is affected by the world around you.

Be Connected

Visit our Web site

If you enjoyed reading this book and are interested in other writings by Doctors Madison and Christine Spurlock, visit our Web site at spurlockchiropractic.com.

If you're interested in finding out more about how Doctors Madison and Christine Spurlock work or want to become a patient, visit spurlockchiropractic.com.

For Doctors

If you'd like to learn a great way to stay connected with your existing patients and find new patients, educate and empower your community, and position yourself as a health-care expert, visit our Web site at spurlockchiropractic.com.

BUY A SHARE OF THE FUTURE IN YOUR COMMUNITY

These certificates make great holiday, graduation and birthday gifts that can be personalized with the recipient's name. The cost of one S.H.A.R.E. or one square foot is $54.17. The personalized certificate is suitable for framing and will state the number of shares purchased and the amount of each share, as well as the recipient's name. The home that you participate in "building" will last for many years and will continue to grow in value.

Here is a sample SHARE certificate:

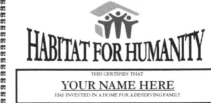

HABITAT FOR HUMANITY

THIS CERTIFIES THAT

YOUR NAME HERE

HAS INVESTED IN A HOME FOR A DESERVING FAMILY

1985-2005

TWENTY YEARS OF BUILDING FUTURES IN OUR COMMUNITY ONE HOME AT A TIME

1200 SQUARE FOOT HOUSE @ $65,000 = $54.17 PER SQUARE FOOT
This certificate represents a tax deductible donation. It has no cash value.

YES, I WOULD LIKE TO HELP!

I support the work that Habitat for Humanity does and I want to be part of the excitement! As a donor, I will receive periodic updates on your construction activities but, more importantly, I know my gift will help a family in our community realize the dream of homeownership. **I would like to SHARE in your efforts against substandard housing in my community!** *(Please print below)*

PLEASE SEND ME _____ SHARES at $54.17 EACH = $ $_____

In Honor Of: _____

Occasion: (Circle One)   HOLIDAY   BIRTHDAY   ANNIVERSARY

     OTHER: _____

Address of Recipient: _____

Gift From: _____ *Donor Address:* _____

Donor Email: _____

I AM ENCLOSING A CHECK FOR $ $_____ PAYABLE TO HABITAT FOR HUMANITY <u>OR</u> PLEASE CHARGE MY VISA OR MASTERCARD *(CIRCLE ONE)*

Card Number _____ Expiration Date: _____

Name as it appears on Credit Card _____ Charge Amount $ _____

Signature _____

Billing Address _____

Telephone # Day _____ Eve _____

PLEASE NOTE: Your contribution is tax-deductible to the fullest extent allowed by law.
Habitat for Humanity • P.O. Box 1443 • Newport News, VA 23601 • 757-596-5553
www.HelpHabitatforHumanity.org

9 781600 376894